REFLEXOLOGY

Explains the techniques of the ancient art of foot massage. In the feet are mirrored all the organs of the body, and this   and drugless way of stimulating them works to r·   ·dy and restore its functi··

REFLEXOLOGY

Techniques of Foot Massage
For Health and Fitness

by

Anna Kaye and Don C. Matchan

THORSONS PUBLISHERS LIMITED
Wellingborough, Northamptonshire

First published in the United Kingdom 1979
Seventh Impression 1985

Original American edition published by
Strawberry Hill Press, San Francisco, California

ISBN 0 7225 0562 0

Printed and bound in Great Britain

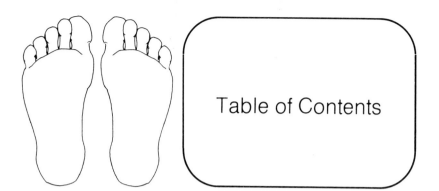

Table of Contents

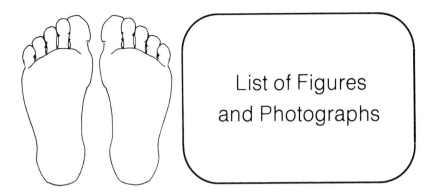

List of Figures and Photographs

Figure:

Photo:

Acknowledgements

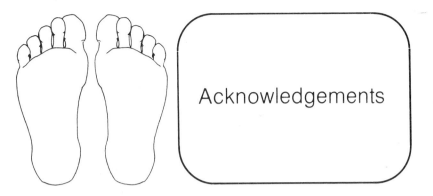

Acknowledgements

Our warm appreciation goes to a bright spirit, a brilliant writer in her own right and an eternally inspiring worker for the good — Betty Gyneth T. Franklin of Fairfax, California. It was she who suggested that the work of Anna Kaye is important, and would make a "good story."

That suggestion was the basis for an article featured prominently in *Let's Live* magazine (444 North Larchmont Blvd., Los Angeles). Titled "Reflexology: It Works," the article was well-received by *Let's Live* subscribers. This book is an expansion of that article, a major revision with important additional material on the secret of "making it work," with many valuable tips for the prospective masseur.

Another of the "weavers," without whom there still would not have been a book, is the widely-known and acclaimed Linda Clark, a long-time contributor to *Let's Live* magazine, and the author of more than 18 books dealing with natural approaches to health. She suggested that this would make an interesting book — and our publisher agrees.

The precision photography is the work of Anna Kaye's talented brother — scientist-inventor Jan Wagner of Oakland, California, who took 80 photos with the assistance of his wife, Jadwiga, who also acted as his "foot model." From these photos we selected the most appropriate for this book.

The sketches and diagrams, orginated by Anna Kaye, were given a professional touch by two budding young artists, Donna Lion of San Francisco and Augie O'Connor of Capitola, California.

Appreciation is also expressed to Mrs. Kaye's highly respected teacher and friend, Dr. F.M. Houston, whose seminars in "Contact Healing" she attended; to Dr. Randolph Stone; to the late Mrs. Eunice Ingham Stopfel, one of the pioneers in this field; and to Mrs. Stopfel's nephew and niece, Dwight Byers and Eusebia Messenger, R.N., who are continuing Mrs. Stopfel's work.

We are grateful, too, to those who encouraged us to do this book, one of whom, Geri Matchan, generously gave up the time she might have spent with her husband so the project could be completed.

And a special note of thanks to Dr. Frank A. Baker of Mankato, Minnesota, whose incredible and unceasing quest for knowledge resulted in valuable source material.

About the Authors

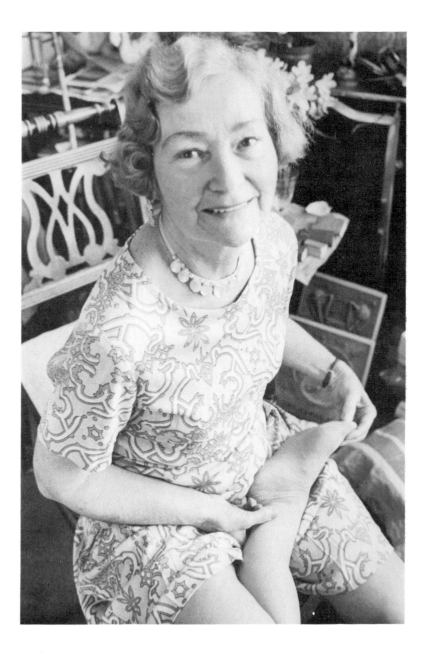

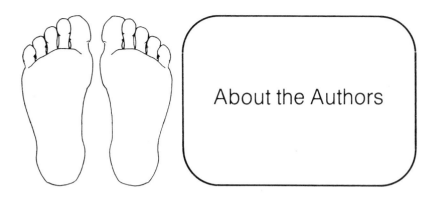

About the Authors

Anna Kaye was a World War II refugee from Poland, where her late husband, Leon Kaye, was a member of the advisory board for the President of Poland, representing the Ministry of Justice. Mrs. Kaye was an attorney-at-law in Lwow (East Poland).

Anna Kaye surprises people when they learn that she is 72 years of age. Her photo for this book, taken two years ago, tells more eloquently than words that she practices what she preaches. She is a healthy human being, physically, mentally, and spiritually.

It has not always been that way however. During the 1940's, she began to lose her sight. She started to learn the Bate's method in Germany and her vision began to improve. In New York, after her arrival from Germany, where she and her husband had been prisoners-of-war, she enrolled in a two-year training course in the Bates' Method, conducted by Clara Hackett, author of *Relax and See*. Mrs. Kaye's vision returned to 20-30, and she decided to teach the method. After 500 hours of practice/teaching, she became a certified instructor in 1954. Shortly thereafter, the couple moved to California.

Anna Kaye's work in eye training led her into a study of reflexology and related areas. She has completed many courses, including those conducted by Dr. F.M. Houston of Pine Valley, California; courses in polarity therapy by Randolph Stone, Ph.D., of Chicago; and a dozen workshops sponsored by a pioneer in the field in this country — the late Eunice I. Stopfel, author of two books on reflexology. She is also familiar with Shiatsu, an Oriental massage technique. Mrs. Kaye has found great value in all of these inter-related disciplines, and in the 14 years in which she has been working with reflex compression massage, she has naturally developed techniques of her own — which she passes on to readers of this book, as well as to those who attend her seminars and workshops. A former student of psychoanalysis in Germany under Prof. G. Schmaltz, a disciple of the great C.G. Jung, she is a psychoanalyst in her own right. And so along with compression massage and the therapy of relaxation, she places heavy emphasis on one's mental attitudes and the control of emotions.

Don C. Matchan, a professional writer and journalist, is Editor of the National Health Federation *Bulletin*. He is also the author of *We Mind If You Smoke* (New York: Pyramid Books, 1977), and co-author, with Phyllis Harrison, of *Helping Your Health Through Handwriting* (New York: Pyramid Books, 1977).

Preface

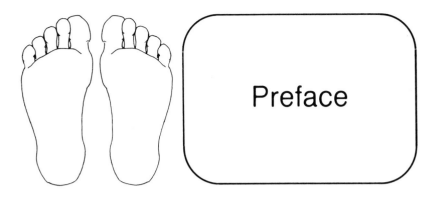

Preface

Like acupuncture, reflexology — the technique involving compression or finger massage at specific points on the feet (or alternatively, the head, hands or body when necessary) — has its roots in antiquity. Reflexology's heritage is that of the Oriental culture, and it is known to have been practiced as long ago as the third millenium B.C. And again like acupuncture, it is gradually becoming "respectable" as a form of therapy for physical disorders ranging from migraine headaches to a sluggish liver or a lethargic pancreas. The basic pattern of energy flow is recognized in all the branches of natural healing — acupuncture, Shiatsu, zone therapy, reflexology, and polarity therapy. The form of compression massage dealt with in this book relies upon the cooperation of natural forces within the body to aid in the process of healing.

More and more, Americans are coming to realize that there is much to be learned from the ancients. If you happen to be one of this breed, if you are reluctant to use drugs, and if you would rather avoid the hospital syndrome — believing that if Nature can create such a perfectly synchronized and delicately balanced apparatus as the human body, then perhaps a "natural" approach to healing makes sense — then you will find it worth your time and concentration to familiarize yourself with the techniques described here — for your own use, and of course to help others, if you are so inclined.

Containing the most detailed description of the technique yet to be published, this book is a guide for everyone, written so all may take advantage of this ancient and wonderful science.

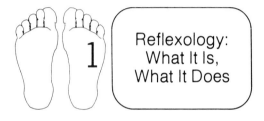

1 Reflexology:
What It Is,
What It Does

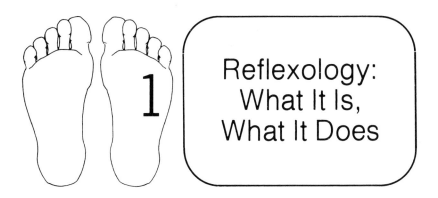

Reflexology: What It Is, What It Does

Reflex: "an involuntary response to a stimulus . . . which is specific and predictable. . ." —*Taber's Cyclopedic Medical Dictionary*

The January, 1973 issue of *Vogue* magazine described the principle that makes reflexology work as "a theory which boils down to this: There are channels of energy coursing through the body; each important organ and muscle is connected by a network of nerves to a tiny point on the foot where the energy terminates. As circulation in the feet slows down — through illness, wearing shoes, or lack of exercise — crystalline deposits form at the nerve endings. By deep-compression foot massage, the deposits are broken up, encouraging the whole body to keep perking along at peak efficiency."

Several thousand years ago, perhaps as long ago as five millenia, the healing arts still employed natural methods. Practitioners of the healing arts (priest-doctors) in the Oriental cultures discovered that life-sustaining energies circulate in the human system; too, how this circulation is linked to the function of internal organs. They learned empirically the location of areas and points, and how manipulation of them could be used to restore circulation when stagnation occurred or energy pathways were blocked. Clearing the energy pathways resulted in the restoration of vitality, balance, a disappearance of the symptoms of disease, and a consequent restoration of health.

One of the intricate healing systems developed by the ancients was reflexology, along with the inter-related disciplines of zone therapy, polarity therapy, acupuncture, Shiatsu, etc. The traditions of this science and teaching have fortunately made their way to the West, where they are gradually winning acceptance.

Reflexology is based on the knowledge of how to accurately manipulate the body's intricate stimulus-response mechanism. But its successful application depends upon three factors: (1) communication, (2) cooperation, and (3) coordination.

Communication is fundamental to the universe, and all life within it. As part of the universe, we are in constant communication with, and influenced by, the surrounding environment, not only that of Earth, but of the solar system as well. Many of us have had the experience of physical response to weather conditions, a common example of which is the arthritic arm or knee that warns a change is due. Earl J. Livingstone, a naturopathic doctor writing in the February, 1975 issue of *Herald of Health* (Mount Ayr, Iowa 50854), said that weather influences the autonomic nervous system, which in turn can "trigger disease and cause circulatory disorders." Body weight can also be influenced by reactions to weather — reportedly as much as a five pound increase is possible between morning and night. (This is not an excuse for overeaters, however!) Certainly the body is marvellously sensitive and adaptable, and as a balancer of the body's energies, reflexology has a major role.

A universe is defined as a "self-inclusive system characterized by order and harmony." (Webster's) We can think of our body as a small cosmos, conceived as an orderly system, a harmonious unit. These two essentials — order and harmony — are possible within the human system *only when there is cooperation and coordination among the organs.* Thus was our system originally devised by a higher authority.

Within the organism, communication is incessant — maintained through a complex system of blood circulation, circulation of energy currents from cell to cell and between the organs via the nervous system, and electromagnetic, vibratory exchange between body and mind. This vital energy, termed by Bergson the "life-force," circulates in a balanced, rhythmic way between all the organs, permeating every living cell and all tissue. This life-sustaining energy flows through surface as well as subcutaneous and deep-seated tissues. It follows predictable patterns or paths, about which you will be learning in this book.

A reflex is an involuntary response to a stimulus; more particularly, it is a reflex-action of an organ, muscle, or gland, reached by the energy current initiated by a stimulus. Reflexes are specific, predictable, and purposeful.

The reflex response of an organ can take place only if the neural pathway between the point of stimulation and the responding organ is intact, with no blockage, or if the pathway can be cleared forcibly by a passing impulse. Known as a reflex arc, this neural pathway passes through neurons, which are actually the nerve cell, the structural and functional unit of the nervous system. Its main function is to conduct impulses initiated by stimuli.

By pressing certain points on the feet, we are starting "afferent impulses." The term "afferent" means to bear or conduct inward toward the center. Messages are given to the nerve cells called afferent neurons, and they in turn transmit them inwardly into the body to the central stations. The impulses coming from the feet *do not* reach the spinal cord. Rather, they are directed by other neurons in the prevertebral ganglia. These neurons are called "efferent neurons" ("efferent" means to carry away from the center toward the periphery), which perform the function of conveying the impulses *out* from this point to the corresponding organ, muscles or gland. The ganglion is a mass of nerve cells located outside of the spinal cord or brain. This explains why impulses started from the pressure points on the feet do not cross to the other side of the body, but travel in vertical zones and reach the organs on the same side of the body. These responses are incorporated into the autonomic nervous system, the division of the nervous system that regulates primarily interior and involuntary action, as of the intestines, heart, and glands.

Compression massage deals with subcutaneous receptors located deeper than the skin, that is, not in the skin, but reaching them through the skin.

What is a stimulus? It is any agent or factor able to evoke response in the organism, even inducing a physiological change. In our work, stimulus means contact and pressure which initiates an impulse or message transmitted through the nerve fibers. The stimulus has a direct influence on protoplasm, the thick, viscuous, colloidal substance constituting the physical basis of all living activities — assimilation, growth, secretion, motility, irritability, reproduction. Protoplasm makes possible muscle contraction and gland secretion. It is interesting to note that it is only comparatively recently that scientists have been able to prove that a nerve impulse causes a muscle or an organ to react through indirect stimulation. Thus the entire process of involuntary reflex action is transmission of a message *inwardly* from a receptor to a nerve center, and *outwardly* to a particular muscle or gland.

To recapitulate: Pressure applied to a nerve ending constitutes a "stimulus." This stimulus sets in motion a "nerve impulse," an electro-chemical impulse which effects a change in nervous processes. (It is *not* a flow of electricity. Nerve impulses travel at the rate of about 270 miles per hour, while electricity travels at the speed of light.) When pressure is applied at a specific point, the impulse passes through afferent neurons to the clump of neurons standing outside the spinal cord, which are known as "ganglia." In the ganglia, the impulse contacts intercalated neurons. Here the message is taken over by efferent neurons and the impulse then travels via efferent neurons to the particular organ, causing its response: the reflex action.

Our bodies are an "electrochemical plant," literally in motion throughout the day and night. We know that all living activities of the human system depend on protoplasm, and that contraction and relaxation is essential to vitality, and to life itself. The blood vessels, too, must be resilient, able to contract and relax automatically if they are to remain functional. Reflexology teaches that every organ, every gland, depends for its survival upon this ability to contract and relax. When an obstacle is placed in the energy channel — as when acid crystals, wastes, or unused calcium deposits form on the delicate nerve endings of the feet — the energy flow is impeded, and the organ it serves is then affected adversely. The degree to which it is affected depends of course upon the duration and extent of blockage.

Unless a foot is covered with oil, the sensitive fingers and thumbs of a masseur can feel these deposits. Under a steady pressure, they are broken up as a similar pressure would break up a sugar lump. The crystals are then eliminated through the blood stream, urine, or sweat glands. Freed from blockage, nerve impulses complete their circuits, and the organ — unless it has been destroyed by disease — regains ability to function as Nature intended.

Some of the many kinds of *reflexes* are listed below:

Superficial (cutaneous): resulting from contact with the skin.

Subcutaneous: activated by contacting deeper layers.

Conditioned: acquired by training.

Unconditioned: innate; natural or inherited.

Crossed: stimulation on one side of the body causing response on the other side.

Postural: resulting in maintenance of posture.

Antagonistic: reflexes initiated simultaneously at various points, and causing opposite effects.

Allied: reflexes initiated by several stimuli simultaneously at different points, sometimes far apart, which follow the same final pathway, reinforcing each other.

Autonomic: instead of traveling through the central nervous system, afferent impulses enter the prevertebral nerve ganglia from whence they pass to the efferent neurons. These impulses do not cross. Autonomic reflexes are highly complicated ones involving involuntary operation of internal organs. While not fully understood by science, their value as vehicles for amazing healing effects has been amply demonstrated.

Working on the feet, we deal almost exclusively with autonomic reflexes. In the autonomic nervous system, the pathways along which stimuli and impulses travel run vertically through the feet and body (Fig. 1).

Knowledge about reflexes is useful because there may be unexpected occasions when you contact other than autonomic reflexes, such as crossing reflexes, or conditioned ones. While you are working on the left foot, for example, the recipient may suddenly announce, "I felt a 'pinch' on my right side!" This is an indication that for some reason, the reflex crossed. Another time you may detect, by tissue congestion, a dense accumulation of crystals — which you will learn to recognize by touch. Aware that such a spot is normally extremely tender, you might ask whether it is or not. If you are told that that place is never tender, then probably you have encountered a conditioned reflex point. As you become more familiar with reflexes, the results of your work will improve.

Note: We use abbreviated terms when explaining links between points on the feet and the corresponding organs. Instead of saying, "Pressing on this point causes a reflex response on (a specific) organ," we simply say, while identifying the place on the foot, "This reflexes to. . . ." There are more than one hundred "reflexes" in the hands, head and body, and we can use them in addition to, or instead of, those on the feet when massag-

Body Zones

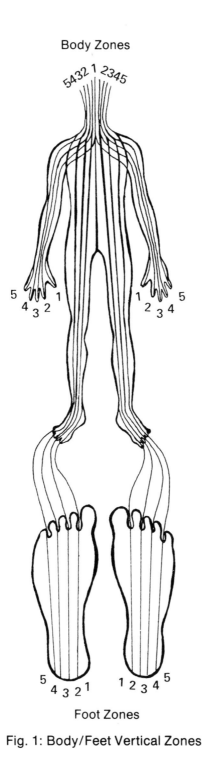

Foot Zones

Fig. 1: Body/Feet Vertical Zones

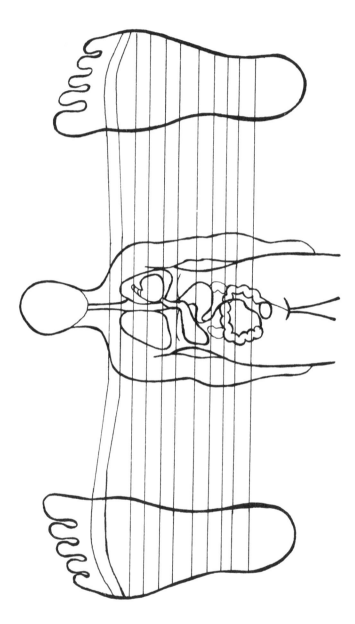

Fig. 2: Level of Reflexes on the Feet

ing certain areas on the feet is either not advisable or impossible.

Let's consider for a moment the intriguing question, "What makes the stimuli and impulses travel through the system in certain specific ways?" The answer to that question is the law of polarity. All that exists — every atom, every cell, the entire system — possess two poles: electric, magnetic, or positive-negative. Poles are the extreme points of an axis, with opposite physical qualities. The ability to exist depends upon forces of interaction between the two terminal points. This interaction is circulation of energy, and it is taking place constantly.

The human system functions in accordance with the law of polarity. Tradition teaches — and experience confirms — that the key points are the head and the feet. They constitute the poles between which ten separate energy currents circulate — five in each half of the body between the head, the five toes, and the five fingers (Fig. 1). These currents flow in perpendicular, meridian-like lines, called zones. They can be contacted — particularly successfully — at their terminal points. The zones of the hands converge at the shoulder area with the rest of the vertical zones.

With the center vertical line marking Zone 1, zones then extend toward the periphery through anterior and posterior portions of the body. Thumbs and big toes represent Zone 1, little toes and little fingers, Zone 5. The soles of the feet correspond with the palms of the hands. Each zone includes all organs through which it passes. And each half of the head and big toe contains the five zones, besides comprising the principal zone-Zone 1.

Pressing (stimulating) points on the feet evokes polarity reflexes in all the organs in a particular zone. Massaging reflex points in the various zones benefits one's health because of the resultant polarizing and balancing of vital energies. Stimuli and impulses sent from the feet remove blockages and stagnation which prevent the natural flow of vital energy.

The vertical zones are also pathways of the gravitational force. Opened by traveling impulses, the neural pathways relax, and troubled organs improve. An organ may be underactive or overactive. Normalizing energy circulation normalizes blood circulation, resulting also in increased activity of the underactive organ, or in inhibited activity of the overactive organ.

The horizontal levels at which you can reach reflexes via foot massage can be determined by referring to Fig. 2 — a diagram showing the position of organs in relation to horizontal levels on the foot.

In addition to the zone pattern, there are other polarity patterns that cross and overlap without interfering with each other's work. The left side and the right side of the body represent two lateral poles. Smaller lateral poles also exist: center, upper, and lower.

Memorize and retain in your memory the image of the zone pattern and the location of organs. You can learn more about this fascinating subject through the books of Dr. Randolph Stone, *Vitality Balance,* and *Polarity Therapy.* These polarity reflexes may be worked on if there is a good reason for not working, or besides working, on the feet.

The head contains many specific reflexes. Cranial bones are inter-laced by a fibrous tissue capable of hinge-like action to allow expansion and contraction of the brain in its rhythmic motion. Contacting points on the head stimulates responses in related energy fields. Even light pressure is helpful. Sore spots indicate stagnation and blockage. All body areas, and functions, are represented in the brain — the generating plant for the entire nervous system. The brain receives messages from every part of the body and mind and relays messages to organs. It is a miraculous system, indeed! Impulses activated by pressure (or contact) points on the head act through the skeletal system.

Obstructions in energy lines and fields register as pain, or in certain conditions as limitations in motion and function, e.g., a stiff neck or a pain-ful back. Energy blockage also interferes with blood circulation, usually first noticed in the extremities. Feet or hands may become stiff, cold, and often painful. Waste products accumulate at the lowest point of gravity — sediment in the form of tiny lumps and crystals which can be distinctly felt under the thumb and fingers as you work on the feet (do not use knuckles for pressure). This is why there is *no substitute* for the human hands. No machine can give you this information.

If you sincerely want to help others — or yourself for that matter — then you must sense where to concentrate, learn how much pressure to use, and determine which organ or organs need the most help. We know that if one organ is not functioning properly, others may also be affected. Study anatomy and physiology. When you know which organs are related more closely to each other, you will work not only on the problem organ, but also on associated ones. No machine can give you this information — only the extremely sensitive tips of the thumbs and fingers. When sedi-ment and crystalline deposits are crushed by pressure, the blood removes them, allowing energy currents again to reach the end-point in the extremities, and thus be "grounded." In this way the harmony-polarity balance is reestablished in the system. This type of massage *cooperates* with the natural forces of the body.

Tension causes energy stagnation and blockage, a condition quickly spotted when pressure is applied — you are liable to get an "ouch!" As the condition improves with massage, the pain lessens, even during applica-tion of pressure. Please understand, however, that *tenderness does not necessarily indicate that organs are sick.* In the foot of a healthy person, tenderness indicates a high level of tension. There will be improvement with the relaxing effect of massage, but how long it lasts depends on the recipient's mental attitude and whether or not the mind is constantly creating new problems. Other elements to be considered are diet and eating habits, his or her work situation, personal relationships, amount of sleep, and still other factors. So it is hardly possible to answer the ques-tion so often asked, "How long will it take to improve?" No two persons are identical, and very few are even similar. And even with the same person, a particular method may work in a different way at another time. Composi-tion of the air, altitude, time of years, the weather — even the time of day — exert significant influences on the body and mind.

To obtain what the masseur and recipient would term good results if the condition is chronic, requires more time of course than in an acute condition like a cold or the flu. Almost immediate relief is possible in acute conditions — not for everyone, though we would estimate that four or five can be helped.

IN SUMMARY:

Reflexology performs the following functions:

1. Removes waste deposits from the feet, permitting grounding of energy.

2. Removes congestion and blockages from the energy pathways, permitting unobstructed flow of energy through the organism.

3. Balances polarity.

4. Improves blood circulation.

5. Normalizes organ and gland function, activating or inhibiting their performance, thus improving the cooperation and coordination of organs.

6. Relaxes the whole system, even the mind, in an "uncanny way," as the late Eunice Ingham Stopfel said.

It is generally conceded that 75% to 80% of the ailments common to much of mankind are caused by tension. Strain, stress, and tension are not natural conditions, and distressing effects are felt throughout the system when subjected unduly to them. Relaxation is a prerequisite to health.

References:

Dr. Randolph Stone, *Polarity Therapy, Vitality Balance, Energy,* available from Dr. R. Stone, 7557 South Merrill Ave., Chicago, Ill. 60649, or Dr. Pierre Pannetier, 401 North Glassell, Orange, Calif. 92666

Eunice Ingham Stopfel, *Stories the Feet Can Tell,* and *Stories the Feet Have Told,* Ingham Publishing, P. O. Box 8412, Rochester, N. Y. 14618

Dr. Joe Shelby Riley, *Zone Reflex,* Health Research, Lafayette St., Mokelumne Hill, Calif. 95245

M.D. Chesney, M.D., *Zone Therapy Is Scientific,* Health Research (above)

Dr. F.M. Houston, *Contact Healing,* and *The Healing Benefits of Acupressure,* Keats Publishers, Inc., New Canaan, Conn. 06840

F. T. Bailey, *Zone Chiro,* pub. by author, Salt Lake City, Utah

Taber's Cyclopedic Medical Dictionary, F. A. Davis Company, 1915 Arch St., Philadelphia, Pa. 19103

Arthur J. Vander, James H. Sherman, and Dorothy Luciano, *Human Physiology,* McGraw-Hill Book Company, 1221 Avenue of Americas, New York, N. Y. 10036

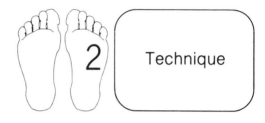

2 Technique

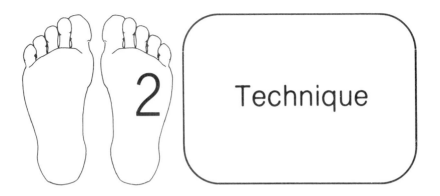

2

Technique

Compared with the rest of the body, the feet are small. Yet their importance cannot be measured by that criterion. In addition to their role of providing mobility, they are a treasure house, harboring all of the nerve endings which make it possible to establish contact with every organ and gland in the body. The pinhead size points on the foot, which connect with the body's internal mechanism, are situated very close together. Larger organs are represented by a larger corresponding area on the foot.

When we give an overall reflex compression massage on the feet, not even the most minute point should be omitted. Every point of about 1/16 of an inch corresponds to, or is linked to, one part of a specific organ or gland. Failure to apply pressure to that point means we may miss the very place most in need of help.

By using the specific technique described here, and by applying it systematically and consecutively to the areas described elsewhere in this book, we achieve complete coverage of all reflexes, and get the results we seek.

The "technique" as used in this context, is a particular way of holding and moving the thumb. Before working on yourself or anyone else, master

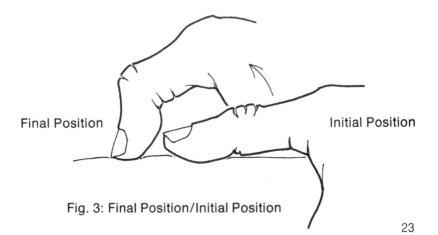

Final Position   Initial Position

Fig. 3: Final Position/Initial Position

it. It is quite simple, really. Here is what might be termed a slow-motion description of how to go about it:

Place your thumb flat on the foot. Then slowly bend it until the portion of your thumb from the tip to the first joint reaches a vertical position (i.e., a 90° angle) in relation to the foot surface. In this position (Fig. 3), apply the pressure straight in, without moving the tip of your thumb forward, backward or sideways.

One of the reasons for applying pressure to the points on the foot is to

SIMPLIFIED   DIAGRAM OF INTERNAL   ORGANS

ANTERIOR   VIEW

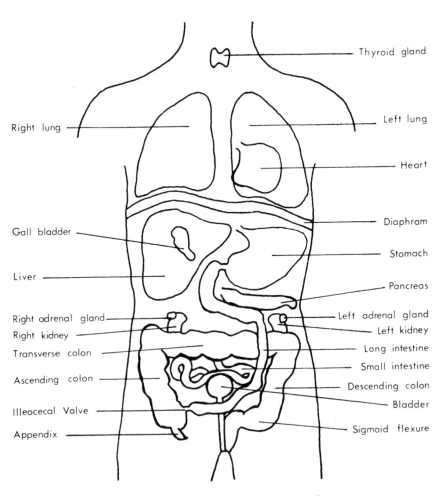

Fig. 4: Simplified Diagram of Internal Organs

crush the crystalline waste deposits which have accumulated at the nerve endings, pulverizing them so that they can be carried away by the blood to points of elimination. If your thumb does not remain constant at the point of pressure, but slips or glides even slightly, you miss the reflex point and pull the skin over the deposits instead of crushing them. Even if deposits are partly broken up in a gliding motion, it is a cardinal principle of reflex compression massage that the pressure on a given point is the stimulus initiating the impulse which travels through the zone and reaches each organ in the zone. This results in the completion of the reflex response. Thus, the points must be precisely pinpointed. So please remember: the pressure point is *not* the gliding point.

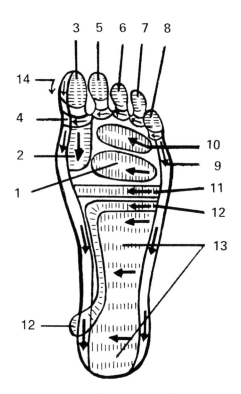

Fig. 5: Foot Diagram (Sequence of areas to work on)
(Same sequence applies on right foot)

Pressure is to be maintained for only an instant, and is then released by straightening the thumb. The thumb is again placed in the flat position on the skin's surface for another moment, after which it starts to bend again to 90° on another pressure point. This movement of alternately bending and straightening the thumb moves it forward in tiny steps, making contact with

25

pressure points about 1/16 of an inch from each other. The motion should be continuous, smooth, without jerks, and always in a forward direction — the tip of the thumb should move ahead in the direction in which it is pointed when flat on the skin. Backward motion burns the skin and is only useless rubbing of the skin. This thumb movement might be likened to a crawling caterpillar, and this term — "caterpillar walk" — is used in other chapters.

The direction of the motion should also always be from top to bottom, that is, from the toes toward the heel, or if moving horizontally across the foot, from the outside edge toward the inside. If the direction was reversed, working from the inside to the outside, the toxins from the crushed deposits would be pushed to the extreme end of the foot, making it more difficult to be flushed out by the blood.

Work slowly, so the stimuli do not follow one after the other like shock waves.

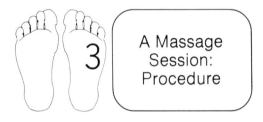

3

A Massage
Session:
Procedure

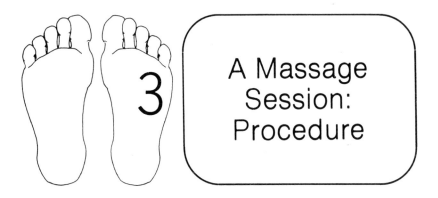

3

A Massage Session: Procedure

The person about to receive a massage may be lying down or sitting, whichever is more convenient. It is important that both the masseur and the recipient, particularly the recipient, be totally comfortable, but not slumped. If the spine is even slightly bent, it creates interference with the flow of energy currents and circulation.

If the recipient is lying on a couch, it must be firm, keeping the spine straight. A thin pillow may be placed under the head, but only if this does not raise it enough to bend the neck. The spine from the hips to the top of the head must remain straight. The feet should rest on a folded towel or thin, soft pillow.

Seat yourself on a chair, facing the recipient, whose feet must be at a level — not too high, not too low — at which you can work comfortably, and at a height at which you can apply the correct angle of the thumb and/or fingers to the feet. The angle is important — even decisive — for reaching the reflexes. The best level is when the tips of the big toes are about at the level of the masseur's shoulders, an inch or two lower perhaps, but no more. (Photo 1)

If the recipient is sitting, the chair must be firm, and comfortable. A straight armchair with soft upholstery is excellent. The recipient should sit straight, with the back vertical, but *relaxed,* not stiffened. Otherwise, the gravity force cannot flow in a natural course, and impulses sent from pressure points will be obstructed. If there is pain or sensitivity in the coccyx (the "tailbone" at the end of the vertebral column), a pillow must be used to sit on, in order to relieve the pressure and to insure comfort. The recipient's legs are outstretched on a stool, at the height of the chair seat, with the knees straight but not stiff. If it proves too difficult to sit with both legs stretched out, one leg can be lowered to the floor while you work on the other foot, and vice versa.

Massage *always* starts on the *left* foot. The human system, as with all creation, functions in conformity with the pattern of polarity. The left side of the body is "magnetic," receptive, and receiving. It readily accepts and transmits stimuli sent from pressure points on the feet. Additionally, a major portion of the lymphatic system — the thoracic duct — is on the left

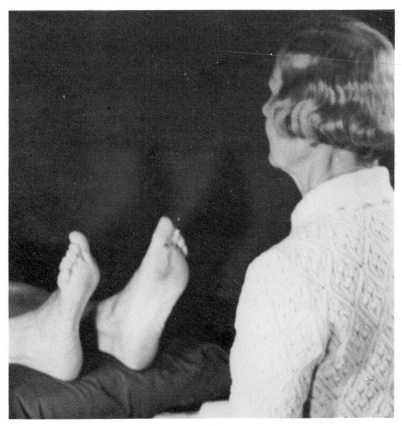

Photo: 1. Feet level

side. Since one of its functions is to halt the spread of unfriendly bacteria and toxins, more toxic residues accumulate on the left side of the body, from where they must be eliminated. Reflex massage helps to accomplish that job.

The right side of the body is the "electric," active, giving, outgoing side, and if compression massage is started on the right foot instead of the left, there is some possibility it will try to reject the stimuli sent from the feet, thus making your work less effective.

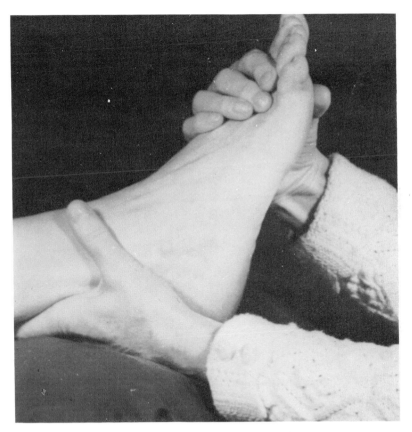

Photo: 2. Position for rotating foot

Observe the expression on the recipient's face. If there is tension expressed there, do not start pressing the reflex points, but first apply relaxation techniques. Gently rotate the foot clockwise and then counter-clockwise. This relaxes the foot and the leg muscles, and the relaxed feeling that comes with the removal of tension spreads throughout the body. With one hand, hold the leg in a stable position by supporting the ankle, so that the upper muscles do not move, while rotating the foot with the other hand. (Photo 2)

Other relaxation techniques:

(a) Rotate the big toe gently, slowly, while holding with the other hand the area slightly below the second joint (where the toe is attached to the foot) in order to stabilize the foot. Rotation of the big toe relaxes the neck and shoulder muscles, where tension frequently accumulates.

(b) A useful technique to relax the feet (and the recipient) is achieved by "stretching" the bones in the foot. With a clenched hand pressing the ball of the foot, and the other hand flat across the top and partly covering the toes, push or press your hands toward each other. This spreads tissues and creates distance between the bones. (Photo 3)

(c) Still another relaxation technique is to gently rub the ankle with both hands, using a simultaneous rotary motion with the palms of each hand. This induces a pleasant feeling of warmth. (Photo 4)

(d) A fifth technique is to rub several times with the "heel" of your palm the inside edge of the foot (corresponding to the spine). Stabilize the foot with your other hand so it is not pushed sideways or bent. Using gentle pressure, run your hand from the top of the big toe to the heel. (Photo 5)

Do not apply these relaxation techniques one after the other. Use one on one foot before starting massage, then on the other. The remaining

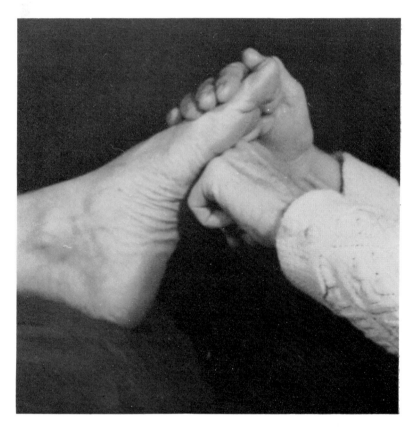

Photo: 3. Loosening foot, "stretching bones"

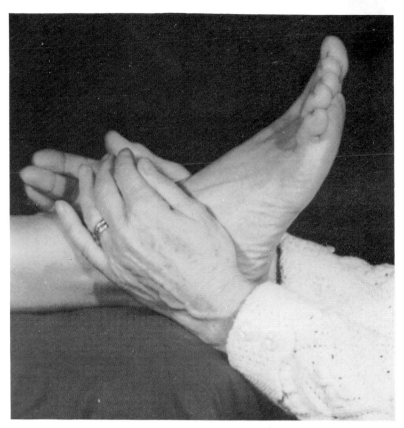

Photo: 4. Rubbing ankle

techniques may be applied during short breaks, after working on areas which are painful. When the session is completed, it is pleasant to perform a few of them as a kind of "dessert" — they make the recipient forget the discomfort and pain that may have been experienced.

Watch the recipient's breathing, because it can give you valuable information. Most of us do not breathe naturally and fully, and shallow breathing is particularly noticeable in tense individuals. How we can breathe is

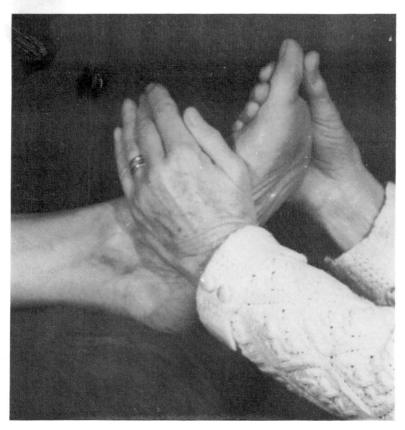

Photo: 5. Rubbing left hand along spine line reflex

extremely important (see Chapter 11, "Breathing"). Among other obvious benefits, correct breathing is a reflex action inducing relaxation. The recipient who does a couple of conscious, full breathings is more able to accept pressure on the feet; and being more relaxed, the recipient will experience less pain. Therefore, do suggest a bit of deep breathing before starting the session.

After studying the chapter, "Technique," explaining how to work, the Foot Diagram (Fig. 5) showing sequence to areas to be be worked on, and the chart showing the location of reflexes (Fig. 15), you are ready to start. The work has to be done systematically and with precision. If not done correctly, some reflexes will certainly be missed and as a result, the work will be less helpful.

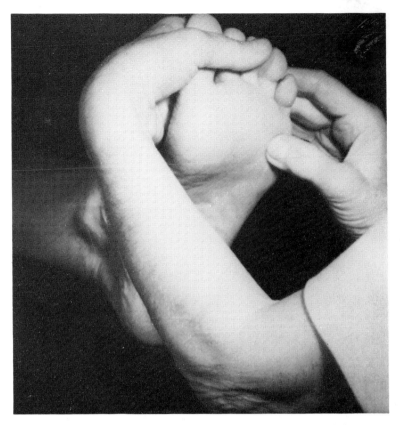

Photo: 6. Starting solar plexus area, right thumb on left foot

Start the massage on the solar plexus area on the *left* foot (Photo 6). With the thumb of your right hand start the "caterpillar walk" from the upper left corner of the solar plexus reflex area. It will be about a half inch or less from the outside edge of the foot. Proceed horizontally across the ball of the foot toward the inside edge. The solar plexus area is marked No. 1 on the Foot Diagram, which shows the sequence of areas to be worked on. To effectively reach the subcutaneous reflexes, gently push the toes away from you with the thumb of your left hand, so that the ball of the foot is more exposed. The surface is also more visible when not wrinkled by pressure.

The fingers of the masseur's left hand are placed (without pressure) on the top of the massaged foot, while the masseur works with the right thumb on the sole, with the fingers of the right hand resting ON the fingers of the

35

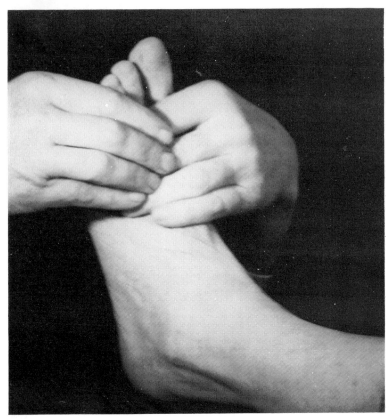

Photo: 7. Fingers resting on the top while working with thumb on the sole

left hand (Photo 7). This prevents pressing simultaneously on the sole and the top of the foot. In some areas, reflexes on the sole and the top of the foot are the same, but others are different, and to press on both simultaneously causes antagonistic or conflicting reflexes, which neutralize each other. So sending reflexes from different places at the same instant is definitely not advisable.

Be sure that the thumb and the fingers of your hand (used to push the toes back and expose the ball of the foot), are not tightly gripping the foot. It would interfere with blood circulation in the toes, causing discomfort to the recipient, thus diminishing the results of the massage.

Proceeding with a caterpillar motion across the ball of the foot (Photo 8), you will reach the indentation extending vertically down from the point between the big and second toe (about two and a half inches down, depending on the size of the foot). At this point, start another path on the solar plexus slightly below the first one, working from *the outside toward the inside* of the foot, across it, and again stop at the indentation and begin

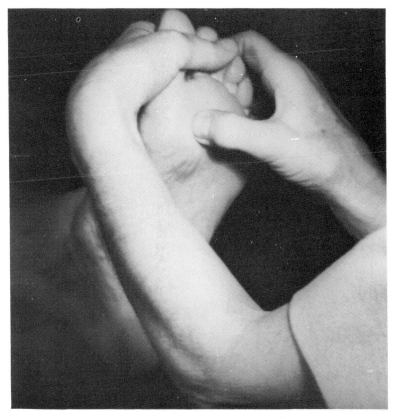

Photo: 8. Last point (right thumb) of first path on solar plexus

a new pathway below the second one. The number of these pathways, whether three, four or five, is determined by the size of the foot. The last pathway is slightly below the ball of the foot.

After covering this area, proceed to the "related" one, No. 2 on the Foot Diagram. This is the ball under the big toe (Photo 9), outlined by the above-mentioned indentation. This indentation, at a point about two to two and one half inches below the starting point (i.e., between the big and the second toe), makes a 90° turn, extending toward the inside of the foot, outlining the section known as the thyroid-related area, (Fig. 6), which includes the indirect reflex to the thyroid. The two reflexes, being partly in the same zone, correspond also to the shoulder blades and to parts of the upper tips of the lungs. With your thumb turned sideways, follow that indentation down, starting from the point between the big and the second toe. By placing your thumb sideways, you reach reflexes located within the indentation.

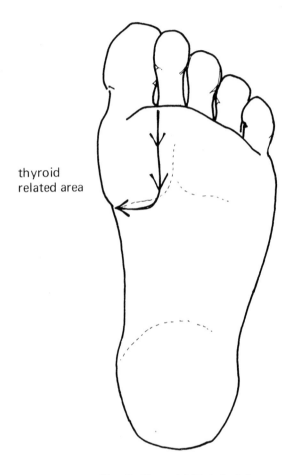

thyroid
related area

Fig. 6: Thyroid-Related Area

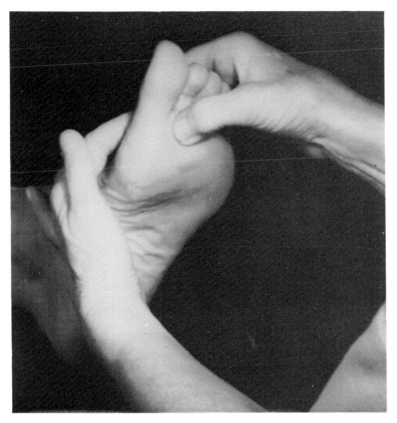

Photo: 9. Starting down, outlining thyroid-related area

Instead of bending and straightening your thumb, keep it bent and move it down along this path with as small "steps" as possible, to the point where the indentation flexes about 90°, extending toward the inside edge of the foot. After changing the motion of your thumb from vertical to horizontal, follow the indentation until you reach the point about a quarter inch from the inside edge of the foot. Keep your thumb sideways, with the thumbnail upward (Photo 10).

Now you are ready to start the pathway from the root of the big toe, (from the point nearest the above-described indentation), doing the caterpillar walk to the point where the indentation flexes toward the edge of the foot. Then do the next pathway, again from the root of the big toe down, a little closer to the inside edge of the foot. Do two, three, or even four of these pathways, again depending on the width of the foot. This covers Area 2 of the Foot Diagram.

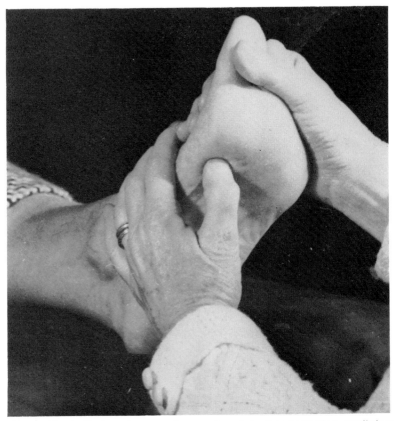

Photo: 10. Left thumb, pressing end point of indentation outlining thyroid-related area

Change now to the right foot, and repeat the procedure. Working through all the areas of the left sole without changing to the right foot would cause imbalance in the circulation of not only the electromagnetic currents, but also the blood, since half of the body would be relaxed, and the other half still tense. This can result in discomfort or slight disorientation. One student told us that while giving a massage before she knew how to alternate the feet, she gave massage on the whole foot without alternating. Then, because the recipient was getting stiff, she asked him to get up for a moment so he could stretch and walk a few steps. On getting up from the chair, he felt so imbalanced that he could not walk upright. He was leaning to one side, and then he stumbled!

Having completed Area 2 on the right foot, return to the left foot for work on Area 3 — the big toe — an important and interesting part of the foot and body. The head is the ruling station or "command post" for the body, and the big toe, at the opposite end of the body, like the head, possesses all five zones. It cannot be explained why this is so, but results and experience confirm it. (Supposedly, it may have something to do with the development of the principal organ system in the embryonic stage.)

The starting point is the top of the left big toe at the edge nearest the second toe (Photo 11). Using the thumb of your *right* hand (because of the angle), proceed down the toe with caterpillar motion to the lower edge of the ball of the big toe. Stop now, and return to the top of the toe and caterpillar walk on the second path, very close to the first one. Repeat three or four pathways, depending on the width of the toe. Be sure that the ball of the big toe is systematically worked through, so no part of the head or brain is missed.

Throughout the time you work on the big toe, it is necessary to support it with the other hand, keeping it stationary regardless of pressure. Neglecting to support the toe diminishes the beneficial effects of the reflex pressure, since movement, involving as it does changing positions and the pulling of muscles, changes the flow of impulses sent from the pres-

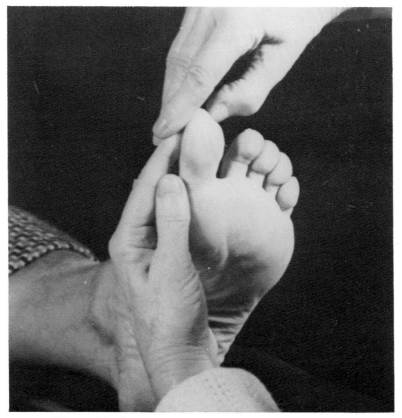

Photo: 11. Starting big toe, left foot, with right thumb

sure points. Note in Photo 12 the correct position of hands in relation to the profile of the foot.

After finishing massage of the ball of the left big toe, work on its root (Foot Diagram — Area 4), starting from the point adjacent to the second toe and "walking" toward the inside edge of the foot (Photo 13). For this pathway, turn the thumb so the nail is down, toward the ball of the foot. Because of the required angle, the right thumb is most effective in stimulating the reflexes to the corresponding parts of the body — the neck and the thyroid gland. Work through this area twice if necessary.

When you have finished the big toe and its root on the left foot, do the same on the right foot. To massage the root of the big toe on the right foot, the *left* thumb may be the most effective. These are not rigid rules — just be certain that your thumb is at the correct angle to the foot (90°).

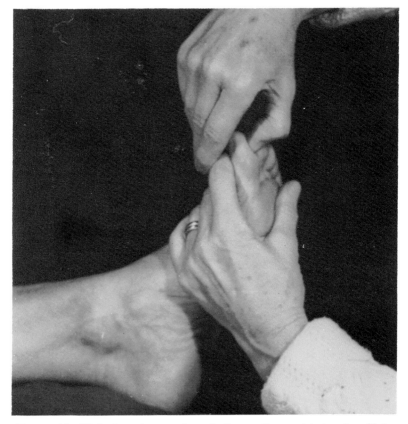

Photo: 12. Right thumb pressing pituitary reflex on big toe (profile)

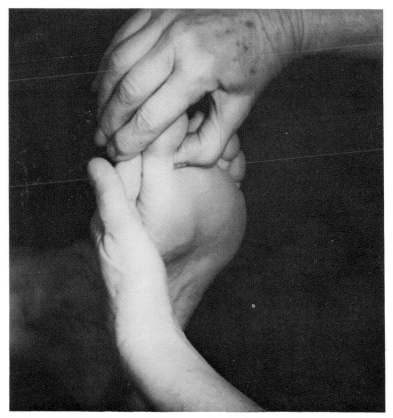

Photo: 13. Right thumb starting root of big toe: reflex to neck and thyroid gland

Now you are ready to work on the toes, second to fifth, on the left foot, and on the pathway on the outside edge of the foot (Areas 5 to 9 on the Foot Diagram). Starting at the upper outside corner of the second toe (Photo 14), work down in a few motions to the end of the ball of this toe. Then do the second path from toe top to the end of the ball, and perhaps a third one, if the width of the toe requires it. Then turn the thumb sideways and work the root as on the big toe. Omit the narrow neck of the toe between the ball and the root, since there are no known reflexes here and the area is often very tender. Perform the same routine on the third, fourth and fifth toes.

We use this sequence of toes, working toward the outside of the foot, because the tops of these toes correspond to the brain, and so it is like encircling it. In addition, the middle of the balls correspond to the sinuses, so you should work on one after the other. Please note that the motion of the thumb is *down* when working on balls, and *toward the inside* when working on roots. The sequence of pathways on each toe is toward the inside of the foot.

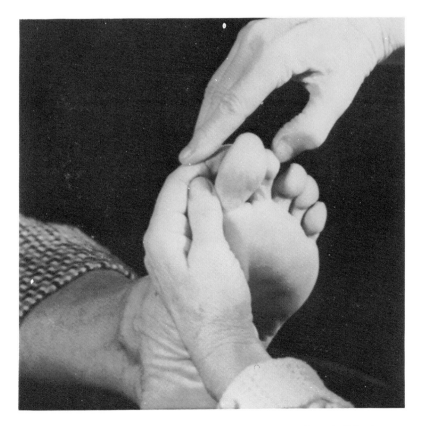

Photo: 14. Starting second toe with right thumb on left foot

Through the fourth and fifth toes (besides the brain and the sinuses), the mastoid, which is related to the ears and the sinuses, can be reached as well. Experience has taught us that the fifth toe of the left foot is also related to the heart. Two persons, who had suffered heart attacks, experienced acute, almost unbearable pain in the fifth toe of the left foot, even while they were lying in bed. Also, a large percentage of persons who have had a heart problem show a high degree of sensitivity when reflex pressure is applied to the fifth toe. Surprisingly, the pain resulting from a heart ailment sometimes is projected to the right side of the chest, and even to the shoulder area on the right foot! The root of the fifth toe reflexes to glands in the armpit, in addition to the ear and shoulder area, where extreme tension frequently accumulates.

After you have completed massaging the root of the fifth toe, work a pathway down toward the heel (Area 9). Follow the line close to the outside edge of the foot (which corresponds to the fifth zone). About two inches from the heel, this line starts to correspond to the sciatic nerve. If it is needed, repeat massage on this line a couple of times. After this area has been completed, change to the right foot and repeat the procedure (Areas 5 to 9).

You are now ready to work on Area 10 of the left foot, starting at the upper part of the ball of the foot, which corresponds to the bronchi, bronchial tubes, and lungs. These reflexes are the same on both feet, but on the left foot it is also the direct reflex to the heart. Complete two or three pathways across this part of the foot, starting from the upper outside corner of the area — about a quarter inch from the outside edge of the foot — and caterpillar walk to the vertical indentation between the ball of the foot and the ball under the big toe. After finishing this area, which is above the solar plexus, repeat the procedure on the right foot.

Area 11 on the *left* foot reflexes to the stomach, spleen (the elongated body behind the stomach), and pancreas. To cover this area, start about a quarter inch from the outside edge of the foot and caterpillar walk hori-

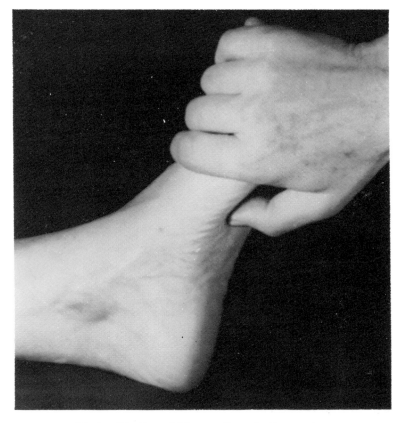

Photo: 15. **From kidney reflex, starting ureter**

zontally toward the inside edge. Stop about a quarter inch from that edge, and repeat a similar path, very slightly below the first one.

Proceed now to Area 12 of the left foot. Start directly under the second path of Area 11, the same distance from the outside edge of the foot, and caterpillar walk across to a quarter inch from the inside edge. At this point, you should have reached the reflex to the kidney and the adrenal gland, a triangular gland situated on the upper surface of each kidney. Now turn your thumb 90° and start to "walk" down along the line parallel to the inside edge of the foot, until you reach the point two to three inches from the heel — depending on the length of the foot (Photo 15). This line corresponds to the ureters, two tubes carrying urine from the kidneys to the bladder. At the point two to three inches from the heel, you probably have reached the end of the ureter. Change the angle of your thumb, and moving horizontally, cross the edge to the oval-shaped area about a half inch above the edge of the foot. Make two pathways about an inch long, with the thumb moving down (Photo 16).

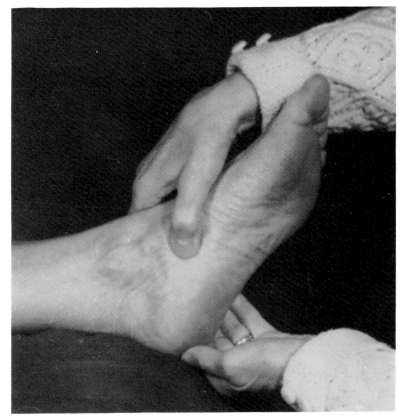

Photo: 16. Right thumb on reflex to bladder

The kidneys, ureters and bladder constitute one unit, functioning together as a unit at all times. For this reason, you should work on each, one after the other, without pause. Among other things, reflex pressure induces relaxation of these glands and organs. Should you massage the kidney area, and ten minutes later work on the bladder, considerable discomfort could result, and if there was tightness or blockage in either ureter or the bladder, it could even be painful. Fig. 7 shows the kidney-ureter-bladder pathway.

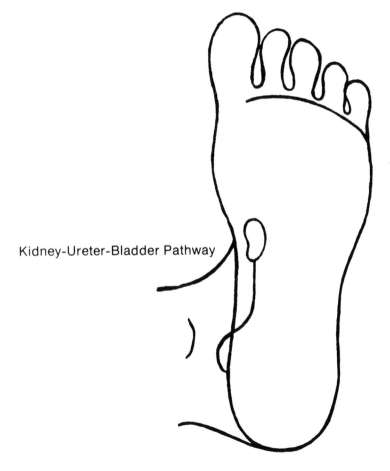

Kidney-Ureter-Bladder Pathway

Fig. 7: Kidney, Ureter, Bladder Pathway

Now we come to Area 13, the large section on the sole of the foot that contains pressure points reflexing to the transverse colon, long intestine, descending colon, small intestine, and the sigmoid flexure of the colon — the lower part of the descending colon near the rectum. All of these organs are closely related and highly coordinated in their functions, so work on them must be completed without alternating to the other foot. Start close to the outside edge of the left foot, at the approximate level of the cuboid bone — the outer bone of the instep — and caterpillar walk horizontally toward the inside edge of the foot. Omit any tendons you may come across. Once again, on reaching a point close to the inside edge, go back to a point about a quarter inch from the outside edge of the foot and start another path slightly below the one just completed. Continue doing pathways horizontally across the foot until you reach the heel.

We are ready now for Area 14 of the left foot. Stabilize it with the left hand, and with your right thumb, starting from the top of the big toe, work down the inside edge of the foot to the heel. This line corresponds to the

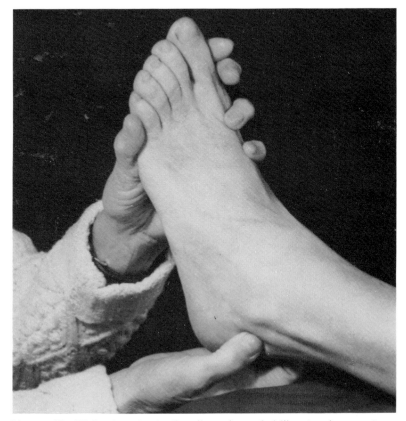

Photo: 17. Right thumb starting line along Achilles tendon: rectum, uterus, prostate, sciatic nerve

spine. When you have finished, you are through with the work on the left sole. You can end up with "dessert": rubbing along this line a couple of times with the heel of your palm creates a pleasant sensation.

Change now to the right foot and perform the same routine to cover Areas 11 through 14, using the appropriate hands for the various positions. On the right foot, the reflexes stimulated are those to the liver, gall bladder, transverse colon, ascending colon, small intestine, ileocecal valve, appendix, right kidney, ureter, and bladder. Although the right ureter is shorter than the left one, it can be reached by massaging through the entire kidney, ureter, and bladder area.

If, during the session, the recipient complains of tender areas, call for a short relaxation break. It may be useful at this point to give a "dessert" massage, and/or stroke the legs gently a couple of times using both hands, with an upward motion only, from the ankle to the knee.

We are ready now to work on the tops of the feet: the outside top, the high top from the toes straight toward the line between the ankle bones and the inside top — in short, the entire foot except for the sole. We start of course with the left foot. With your left hand, lift the foot slightly above the stool, just enough so your right hand fits under the heel (Photo 17). Place the thumb of your right hand slightly above the heel on the outside of the foot, with the index and middle finger at the same level on the inside of the foot. Start moving up, point by point, without skipping any spaces, pressing on both sides along the Achilles tendon. Do not press the tendon itself, just the indentation that runs alongside it. Proceed to a point two or three inches above the ankle bone. This area is related to the rectum, the uterus or prostate, and the sciatic nerve. This is frequently a very tender area, particularly if the condition is chronic. Then massage another pathway parallel to the first one, but a little farther from the Achilles tendon and the edge of the back of the leg. This path more closely corresponds to the sciatic nerve.

The next step is to use the thumb with a caterpillar motion on the outside of the foot, from the heel edge toward the ankle bone. Stop when you are about a half inch or a little less from the ankle bone, and start the next pathway very close to the first one, using the same technique. Do several more, very close to each other. The first few pathways — up to five — should converge toward the ankle bone; the next several extend toward the space between the outside and inside ankle bone (Fig. 8).

The cuboid bone is on the outside edge, at about half the length of the foot. At this point, begin to use the fingers of both hands, supporting the foot on the sole side with the heels of your palms (Photo 18). With extremely small steps, work toward the ankle. Press between tendons and omit the bones. After reaching the fifth toe, the starting points of pathways are at the roots of the toes. Proceed toward the line between ankle bones, keeping the fingers bent. Repeat these pathways until the top of the foot has been covered.

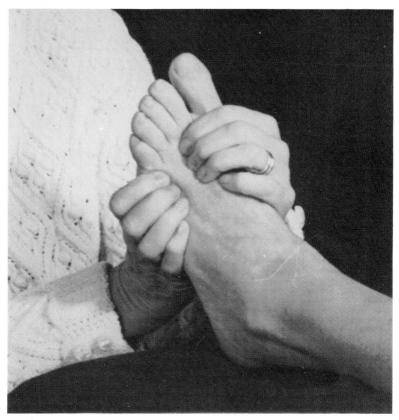

Photo: 18. Both hands between tendons on top of foot

When you come to the inside edge of the foot, use the thumb again, moving toward the inside ankle bone, with the pathways slightly converging (Fig. 9). Some reflexes on this part of the foot are tender in 95 percent of the cases. The tender point on the outside of the foot is halfway between the heel and the ankle bone, which reflexes to the ovary or the testicle. Another tender spot is on the inside, halfway between the heel and the ankle bone, which corresponds to the uterus or prostate gland. For some reason, these points are sensitive even in youngsters. Some reflexes on the top space between the big and fifth toe are the same as on the sole side — they "go through," so to speak. These reflexes are to the lungs, shoulder blades, shoulders, and to some degree, the heart. This part of the foot also corresponds to the lymph glands in the front of the body and in the breasts.

Upon finishing the inside part of the top of the foot — the last pathway from the heel to a quarter inch from the ankle bone — start the next area: the line on the top of the foot, between ankle bones (Photo 19). Using either your thumb or the index and middle fingers together, work from the

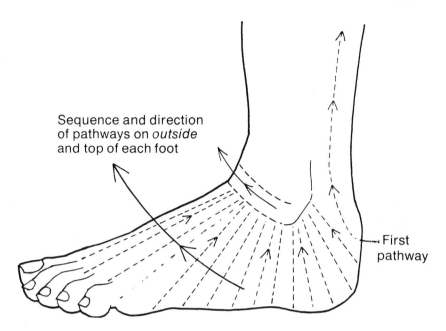

Fig. 8: Sequence and Direction of Pathway on *Outside* and Top of Each Foot

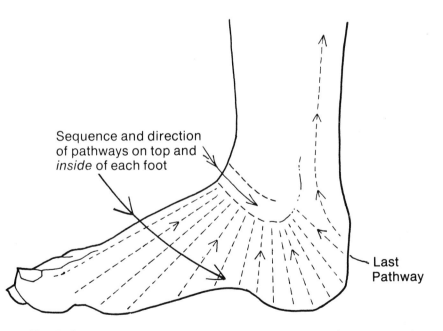

Fig. 9: Sequence and Direction of Pathway on *Inside* and Top of Each Foot

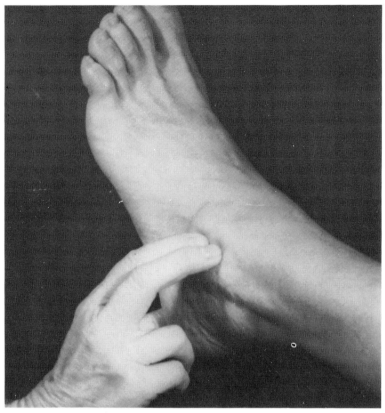

Photo: 19. Starting with two fingers, reflex to groin area

outside ankle bone to the inside ankle bone, which finishes the path. This pathway reflexes to the groin, the lymph glands in the groin, and the nearby fallopian tubes. Fallopian tubes are about four and a quarter inches long and a quarter inch wide and extend laterally from the lateral angle of the uterus to the ovary. Repeat this path two or three times because the lymphatic system is in constant need of drainage.

A particular draining technique, called "milking," is applied for this purpose (Photo 20). Place the thumb in the area between the big toe and the second toe, about an inch below their roots on the sole side, with the index and middle fingers in the same line on top of the foot. Then press and pull toward the toes as if you were milking a cow. Move closer to the toe roots and repeat the motion. The lymph system then clears, drains, and relaxes.

After you have finished all this on the left foot, do exactly the same on the entire top area of the right foot.

When the soles and the tops of each foot are finished, you can go back for brief pressures at places which were particularly sensitive. They will

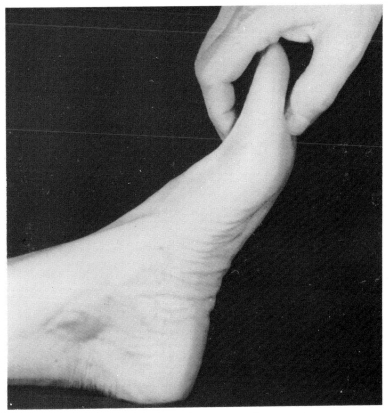

Photo: 20. "Milking," draining lymphatic system

probably be much less sensitive when contacted a second time. Be advised that there are no strict rules stipulating that you should do the repeat massaging — as experience is acquired, you will come to know whether or not it is advisable.

A few points must still be contacted: With your left hand, slightly lift and support the recipient's left foot. With your right thumb, locate by touch — not by pressing — the ankle joint's supporting tendon, which extends from beneath the ankle joint to the toes. Put your thumb below this tendon, near the ankle bone, and press (Photo 21). This point corresponds to the hip area and part of the sciatic nerve. The stimulus is transmitted through the sciatic nerve and its sacral plexus to the rest of the nervous system. This is the reflex connection to the entire nervous system. It is often so sensitive that the recipient jumps up involuntarily, even without application of heavy pressure. *Press only once.* Then go to the same point on the inside of the foot (changing hands because it is nearly impossible to reach it with the right thumb). Next, supporting the *right* foot with your right hand, press the

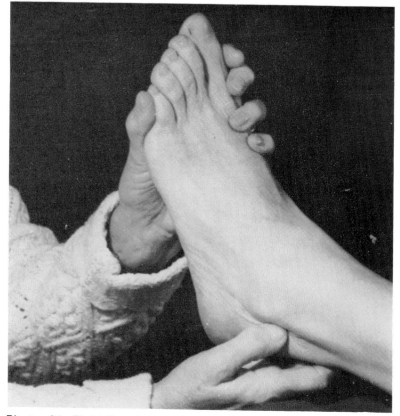

Photo: 21. Right thumb pressing below ankle bone: reflex to hip, sciatic and nervous system

outside point at the ankle bone with your left thumb. Do this also on the inside of the right foot, using the left hand to support the foot, pressing with the right thumb. If the feet are large and heavy, support them by putting the palm of one hand under the heel while you apply pressure with the thumb of the other hand.

It is time now for the exercise called "solar breathing." Contact the lower part of the solar plexus on each foot with the thumbs of each hand simultaneously (Photo 22). Explain in advance what you are about to do and what you expect the recipient to do: slowly increase pressure with the two thumbs while the recipient inhales slowly, taking air down into the abdomen first and filling up from there. When the lungs are full and the pressure of your thumbs is fairly strong, the recipient should hold the breath a second or two while you sustain pressure. Then as the recipient exhales slowly, you gradually release pressure. Inhalation and exhalation are done *through the nose.* Remove your thumbs when the breath has

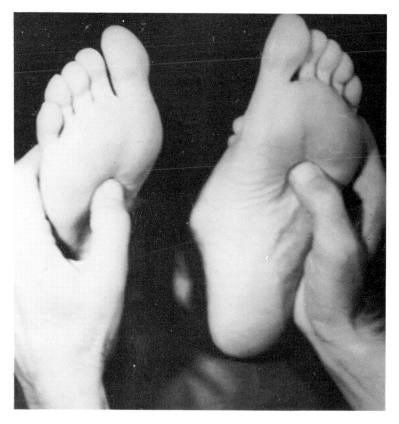

Photo: 22. Both thumbs pressing solar plexus reflex at same time for "solar plexus breathing"

been exhaled. If the recipient enjoys this exercise, it can be repeated up to three times.

The connection between the solar plexus and one's breathing is a vital one. The solar plexus, which is behind the stomach and between the suprarenal glands, is the nerve mechanism servicing most of the involuntary organs. Breathing has a complex physiological effect on these organs and the nervous system. (See Chapter 11, "Breathing.") The combination of deep conscious breathing and sending a stimulus by pressure to the solar plexus, achieves a very special effect: balancing and normalizing the flow of energy through all the pathways from which blockage was removed by the reflex compression massage. You might now suggest that the recipient do a couple of deep yawns — a natural dessert!

This completes the reflex compression massage session. It is not really that difficult, and the more you delve into it the more you will find it fascinating and rewarding — not only for yourself, but for those fortunate enough to have the benefit of your skills.

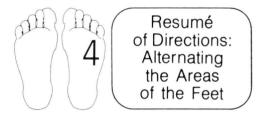

4 Resumé
of Directions:
Alternating
the Areas
of the Feet

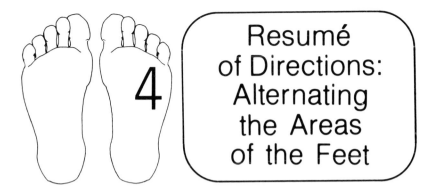

Resumé of Directions: Alternating the Areas of the Feet

1. Start the compression massage on the left foot, doing Areas 1 and 2 on that foot.

2. Change to right foot and do Areas 1 and 2.

3. Return to left foot and work through Areas 3 and 4.

4. Change to right foot and do Areas 3 and 4.

5. Return to left foot and work through Areas 5 to 9.

6. Change to right foot and work through Areas 5 to 9.

7. Return to left foot and work on Area 10.

8. Change to right foot and do the Area 10.

9. Return to left foot and work through Areas 11 to 14.

10. Change to right foot and work through Areas 11 to 14. This completes the work on the soles of the feet.

11. Now work on the tops of the feet: The outside top, high top and the inside part of the top of the feet.

(a) Start at the back of the left foot, slightly above the heel. Proceed along the Achilles tendon (on the indentation behind it) toward the knee, pressing on both sides simultaneously and using the thumb on one side, and the index and middle fingers on the other side, till about two inches above the ankle.

(b) Then start on the outside of the foot, following the pathways converging toward the ankle bone; then work on the top going toward the groin area (line between both ankle bones), pressing with fingers of both hands between the tendons. On reaching the inside edge of the foot, continue working the pathways, using the thumb, toward the inside ankle bone until you reach the back of the heel.

(c) Now work on the reflexes to the groin: the line from outside ankle bone to the inside ankle bone.

(d) Change to the right foot and cover the entire space on top of that foot in the same way as you have just done the left, remembering to *always start from the outside*.

12. Once again on the left foot, press the point slightly below and behind the *outside* ankle bone; then on the same foot press the point beneath and behind the *inside* ankle bone.

13. Change to the right foot and repeat the procedure in the same order.

14. Do not forget "milking": pulling on the middle line between the big and the second toe for drainage of the lymphatic system.

15. Finally — apply the "solar plexus breathing" technique, pressing on the solar plexus area of each foot simultaneously in coordination with the recipient's deep conscious inhalation and then exhalation while releasing the pressure.

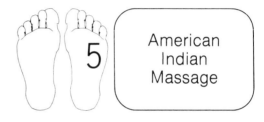

5 American Indian Massage

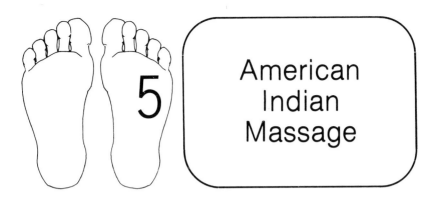

5

American
Indian
Massage

This massage can be administered with or without clothing, although we always prefer to work on persons who are dressed. The recipient should sit on a backless stool in a straight but comfortably relaxed position, with the hands resting a small distance apart on top of a chair-back in front of the recipient. The spine does not have to be absolutely straight and can be at a slightly slanted angle, but the recipient should not be slouched or bent over. (Fig. 10)

First, locate the coccyx. Then position the tips of your thumbs about one half inch from each side of it, and begin to "jiggle" with quick little movements and fairly firm pressure in short steps upwards. When you reach the level of the hips, go back to the coccyx and jiggle once or twice in slanting directions toward the hip bones. When the points about two inches below the hip bones are reached, return to the area of the spine at this level and begin to jiggle upwards. About every eight inches or so, stop for a moment, then continue upwards until you reach the base of the skull, being very gentle on the neck at this point. This upward pressure along the spine directs the life energy upwards from its center in the pelvic area. (Fig. 11) Most people report feeling chills and tingling sensations all over the body.

Having done this, ask the recipient to put the hands on his or her thighs. Then start to manipulate the trapezius muscles (the flat, triangular muscles on the back of the neck and shoulders). Knead them firmly several times, using both hands at the same time on the shoulders.

After doing this, stroke the shoulders, upper arms and back with both hands simultaneously. Proceed gently, without any pressure, from the shoulders down to the waist. This motion helps to spread the energy evenly throughout the body.

This technique is delightfully relaxing, but also invigorating. After it is completed, many people sigh and say that it feels wonderful. In many instances, this massage brings relief from bursitis pain and back pains. The Indian Massage can be given after the foot massage session is completed, as just indicated. There are no strict rules regarding this, and so this massage can be given at any time without having to precede it with a reflexology massage. However, please note that *it should not be done* if the recipient recently incurred a back injury near the "jigging areas" or on the shoulders.

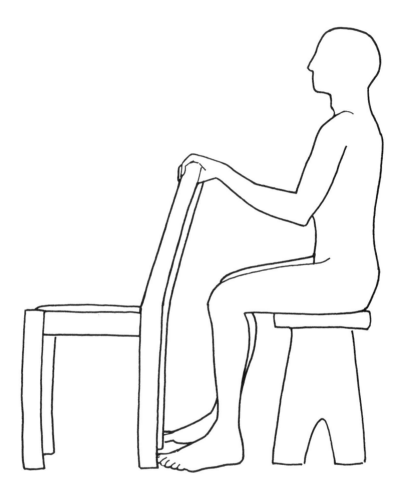

Fig. 10: Indian Massage (Position)

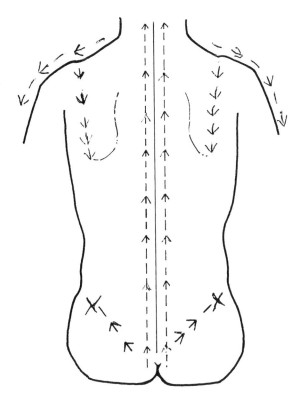

Fig. 11: Indian Massage (Technique)

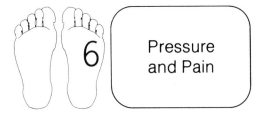

6

Pressure and Pain

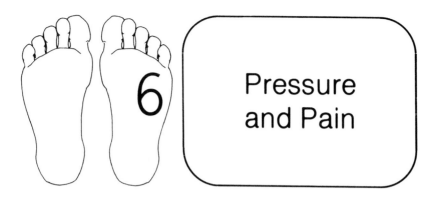

6

Pressure and Pain

In the foregoing chapters, we have explained that effective deep compression massage is accomplished by applying systematic, consecutive pressure to pin–head-size points on the feet. Now the question to be considered is how strong should the pressure be in order to be effective and yet not unbearable.

The pressure should vary according to the physical and emotional/mental condition of the recipient, taking into account also a number of other factors. For a strong, generally healthy person with sturdy skin, who may sometimes go barefoot, the pressure can be quite strong. In cases which are not so obvious, you must make a tentative judgement based upon a careful appraisal. You are usually told why an individual wants your services, and in general what the problem appears to be. Detailed information comes through the observations you make while working on the feet.

One of the first factors to be considered is the condition of the skin. If it looks and feels delicate to the touch, if it seems thin, then the person is sensitive, whether or not that fact is acknowledged. In her book, *New Mind, New Body* (Harper & Row), Dr. Barbara Brown states that the skin can reflect the most subtle indications of a person's emotional state, such as anxiety and apprehension. The skin is a physiological as well as a psychological and emotional mirror of the human being.

Callouses and corns are not necessarily caused by ill-fitting shoes. They indicate as well glandular disturbances resulting from emotional upsets and imbalances. I recall the case of a woman who came to me for massage to relieve tension. During one visit, I found quarter-inch-thick callouses on her feet, though she had none a week earlier! In response to my query as to whether she had had some sort of emotional shock, she said that indeed she had — her marriage had been terminated by her husband who had moved out to live with a younger woman. It had been the most traumatic experience of her life. Fortunately, we do not see this sort of dramatic evidence very often, but it does serve to remind us that the skin reveals the emotional state — and the consequent acute need for relaxation.

So before you start the massage, check the texture, flexibility and smoothness of the skin with your hand. This first feeling and touching of the skin is a prerequisite for a satisfying and successful session. This is why I exclude the use of oils (which are used with some other types of massage) and lotions for compression massage. I advise people not to use lotion on the feet the day of their appointment. Oil or lotion becomes a form of isolation between the recipient's skin and the hand of the masseuse, and causes a gliding effect which results in missing the pin-head-size reflex points.

In this work there is no substitute for the human hand. Electric vibrators and similar types of equipment may be better than nothing, but they are incapable of performing the quality of work possible with human hands. Some of these instruments create an uneven or a jerky stimulus. But there is yet another sound reason for the difference: The body is an electro-magnetic unit. Each cell possesses an electrical charge which radiates outward from, and beyond, the skin's surface. And so it is that this current influences even objects with which the hand comes into contact. Its quality and strength depend on one's physical and mental condition. Reflex compression massage achieves healing in a more subtle way than merely through application of pressure.

Consider all these factors, and *do not work quickly.* It is better to do a thorough job on each foot in one massage than to speed through it two or three times.

Ask the recipient how much pain or sensitivity is being felt, and keep it in mind because this is precious information for you. Pain is a highly complex syndrome, and can be a distressing experience. The terms "low" or "high" "threshold of pain" do not adequately explain the phenomenon of pain. The degree of pain felt depends on the individual awareness and the interpretation given by the one experiencing it. One person announced on arrival that she had "a very low threshold of pain," and asked me to be as gentle as possible. I promised to comply. Her skin was delicate, so at the start of the massage I pressed lightly and gradually increased pressure until it was fairly intense. She indicated that she felt no pain, only the pressure. Her legs were healthy, with no circulation problem, which can diminish the feeling of pain. So I applied strong pressure throughout the session. "How do you feel?" I asked upon finishing. "Just wonderful," she replied. "It was all a very pleasant experience." She did not expect, and thus she did not feel any pain after hearing me promise to use light pressure. I have also had the experience of working with people referred by friends of theirs who told them that this kind of work on the feet hurts. Convinced then that this was a fact, they expected pain, and although young and healthy, it did hurt them. Once again — the power of suggestion!

I had a certain client who, for some reason, was exceptionally sensitive. When the session began, I had barely touched his feet when he began to moan and twist his body. So I experimented: I asked him to close his eyes and told him that I would press the solar plexus area on his foot, and suggested that with his eyes closed he might be able to accept the pressure more easily. He closed his eyes, but I did not press at all. I simply contacted the skin with my little finger. He could not see what I was doing, but the moment I touched his skin he jumped and yelled, "Oh — it hurts!" I then explained what had just occurred, but he did not believe me. This is a rare case, of course, mentioned only because you should be prepared for a variety of reactions, and so that you will always be certain that you do not "torture" anyone by causing either real or imaginary pain. It is better to undertreat than to overtreat. Or, as in the case just described, look for another solution: I informed him that the hands have the same reflexes as the feet, and since it was not possible for him to be comfortable if his feet were being worked on, I would work on his hands. The results were excellent. He relaxed, and at the next session I was able to work on his feet, which now proved much less painful for him.

As Ronald Melzack explains in *The Puzzle of Pain* (Basic Books, New York), pain still is a great puzzle, not fully understood by medical science. It possesses an almost endless variety of qualities. So do not be surprised when one person feels pain for no apparent reason, while another, under similar circumstances and comparable conditions, reports feeling no pain, even with application of considerable pressure.

People's comments can be very interesting. For example, one person might exclaim, "You're hurting me; is it necessary to go through this to feel better?" So you must try to explain why it happens, and what the compression massage is accomplishing. Another may say, "It hurts, but it is a *good* pain." Ordinarily, the pain recedes as an individual improves in health.

Biologically, pain is a signal to the brain that something odd is happening in the system. The receptors (in this case, nerve endings in the skin), the fibers and sensory system transmit neural signals, but they can be modulated by many factors. Perception of pain varies widely among individuals, influenced as it is by biological, physiological, psychological, and even cultural factors. Thus you must consider all these factors, lest, rather than having a productive session, you mistreat the person instead.

Particular care must be used with persons afflicted with such problems as diabetes and such vascular inadequacies as vasculitis. Even if you are not told about such conditions in advance, they are recognizable after the first few moments of massage, or simply by observing the skin. If pinkish in appearance, an unusual color for the feet, start pressing very lightly. If, after pressing several points, the pink color becomes more pronounced, reduce pressure considerably. A diabetic bruises easily, and the bruises may not always heal. This can occur also in the case of vitamin-mineral deficiency, which is frequently the underlying cause of vasculitis — vascular inflammation. Pink-looking feet may indicate such conditions.

Extreme sensitivity in the feet of a normal and healthy appearing person indicates a high level of tension; and if some areas, corresponding specifically to certain organs, are very tender under pressure, it does not necessarily mean that the organ is not functioning adequately. But it does indicate to us that the organ is not functioning optimally because of a blockage of blood circulation and the circulation of energy currents in that zone.

There are exceptions, however. Some individuals with serious health problems do not show even mild sensitivity to pressure. This signals that there is either nerve damage or extremely poor circulation, numbing the feet. Normal sensitivity returns at times following sessions of reflex compression massage.

In connection with the subject of pain, I want to share with you an interesting case history: A man whose leg had been amputated a year earlier made an appointment to see me. During the months following surgery, he had suffered what he described as an almost unbearable pain in the phantom limb. The pain, he said, was not in the remaining portion of the leg near the hip, but in the space where the now severed part of the leg had been — "way down to the foot." Analgesics were not helpful, and the pain was constant, accompanied by an occasional tingling sensation. This is not an unusual phenomenon — about 35 percent of amputees report suffering phantom limb pains. Though not fully explained by science, it is known that while a psychological factor is involved, a subtle physiological action upon the brain is also involved. This gentleman had reached the point where he felt that he might be going insane — how else could he feel pain in a nonexistent limb?

I explained to him that the human body is composed of *several* "bodies." The physical body is material and tangible. The others are composed of much more subtle substances, or vibrations. With a shape identical to that of the physical body, these subtle bodies are present as long as the person lives, overlapping, or rather permeating, the physical body. Esoteric teaching refers to these forms as etheric or astral bodies, and indicates that, among other things, they are connected with, and influence thereby the nervous system, and vice versa. The loss of a limb does not sever or destroy the limb of the etheric or astral body, and the imprint of the injury remains. The pain is transmitted to pain receptors in the physical system, and the conscious mind then receives the message and perceives the pain. He understood this explanation, relaxed, and was ready to accept any help I could give. I worked on his hand, which contains the same reflex areas as the foot, and several times I worked also on the reflexes to the leg. After several sessions, the phantom pain vanished.

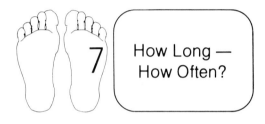

7

How Long —
How Often?

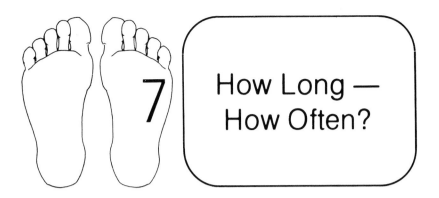

How Long — How Often?

The consideration always arises as to how long at any one time a person should be worked on. As in all things, it varies with every person and circumstance.

One factor is foot size: To administer an exact, systematic massage on the feet of a man wearing a wide size 12 shoe takes considerably more time of course than to give the same thorough massage to the feet of a child or small adult wearing a size 4 shoe.

Another decisive factor to consider is the state of health of the recipient. If a robust individual with healthy feet wants to experience the relaxing sensation produced by reflex massage, and if the feet are not exceptionally tender, you can work up to 45 minutes, or even longer, if the person wants it and is being relaxed by it. On sensitive feet, however, shorten the time. The more painful the pressure is to the recipient, the shorter the time you work, since the pain could very well interfere with one of the primary objectives of reflex massage — relaxation. The session should end considerably sooner for the individual afflicted with a chronic ailment such as diabetes or rheumatoid arthritis. The first session, particularly, should be concluded in 15 minutes, or even less, if circumstances seem to warrant.

In dealing with chronic conditions, invariably there are many crystalline deposits in the feet. They are crushed under the pressure of the reflex massage, and as a result, the toxins from the deposits are released into the blood stream, creating temporarily increased toxicity in the body. The individual will feel quite ill within a few hours, or even a day or two later — a situation which should be avoided if at all possible.

After the first massage session and the ensuing reaction, a better understanding is developed as to how to handle the case — how frequently a massage is advisable, and for how long a period. Generally speaking, a massage can be given twice a week, but in cases of a pronounced reaction, only once a week is advisable, waiting until the effects of a possible reaction have passed. If there is a reaction, it may only amount to the person feeling "a little down" for a day or two.

In the cases involving gall bladder and liver problems, it is usually useful to schedule two sessions a week. If the recipient is a healthy person, and requires relaxation only, it is good to give a daily massage. However, when confronted with an acute condition, such as the flu, you may even work twice a day, but only for short periods. A fever can be broken very quickly by working on the reflex to the pituitary gland for two or three minutes at a time at ten or fifteen minute intervals.

To give an example in which some of these factors were involved: A friend once called me to say that her mother was in bed with the flu, and had a temperature reading of 104°. She asked me what she should do. Recognizing the potential danger — her mother was nearly ninety — I told her to call a doctor at once and to be sure to say that it was an emergency. Her mother refused to do it however, as she was afraid to go to a hospital, and asked me instead to give her a reflex massage. I did so reluctantly, and stayed with the woman for about three hours. After the first whole massage on her feet, I applied pressure to the pituitary reflex at ten-minute intervals. Within three hours the fever had subsided to 99°. She recovered in a few days, which is rare at that age.

This simply emphasizes that *every case must be handled on an individual basis*. This pertains also to the question of how many sessions may be required. Generally, the tenderness diminishes gradually, and if it disappears altogether, further sessions may be unnecessary. We must also take into account the physical and mental condition, the eating habits, and the way of life of the recipient.

An important point: Every generalization can be a gross error. I once met a man at one of Eunice Stopfel's seminars who claimed to be a professional reflexologist. In response to my question as to the length of his massage sessions, he told me that he attempts to "squeeze in" three persons per hour! I did not ask him what percentage of success he had. Apparently he was determined to handle a certain number of cases per day. Do not follow that example. Adjust the length of a session to the individual — not to the clock. The length of a session does not always coincide with the time spent actually working on the feet, because it depends upon how many breaks you need to give between work on painful areas. Also, do give more breaks and "desserts" to a weak or nervous person. It will prolong the session, but not the work itself, and you will be gratified with the more fruitful results.

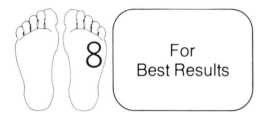

8

For
Best Results

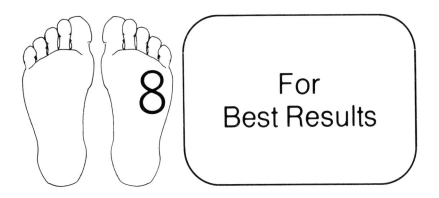

8
For Best Results

Some of the following material was mentioned briefly in Chapter 3. I wish to emphasize, however, some of the things that the masseur should do in order to produce a truly good and effective massage session.

You must see to it that the recipient is sitting comfortably, preferably in an arm chair so that the arms may be in a comfortable position. Some people have a very long coccyx, which may create some pressure there while in a sitting position. Others may be sore from an injury of some sort. Whatever the case may be, if someone is not able to sit quietly for more than a few minutes, supply a proper pillow, and if necessary, allow the recipient to stand up and stretch after working on one area. Massage can also be done with the recipient lying down; this will probably not occur often, but you should be prepared to make adjustment for it when it does occur.

Place a soft towel on the flat pillow on which the recipient's legs are outstretched. Bare legs should be covered with a soft, light material in order to maintain an even body temperature, which aids proper blood circulation.

If the recipient's face indicates tension, try to relax him or her by stroking and rotating the feet, and then gently rotating the big toe. (A doctor once told us that instead of the word "rotation," we should use the term "circumduction," which expresses this particular action more accurately.) Then ask the recipient to consciously loosen his muscles, even if in only one part of the body — the arms and shoulders perhaps. If relaxation is achieved in one set of muscles, the others have a tendency to relax also. Scientists have found that the relaxing of small muscles particularly facilitates relaxation of the whole body.

Suggest a couple of yawns at this point also. Yawning is a natural tranquilizer, a fact unfortunately neglected by most of us in the West. We have all seen animals yawn, but it has even been reported that ants yawn as well!

There is no quick and simple recipe for teaching others how to relax. But we can offer suggestions and explain as we get ready to do the massage that the best results in any undertaking are obtained if we are relaxed. It is simply a matter of economy in the expenditure of energy.

It is important that you too are mentally serene and physically relaxed as you work. The importance of being relaxed in mind and body as you work cannot be over-emphasized. Tension is rigidity. Tense, rigid hands cannot move smoothly, and they may even jerk at times and miss some reflexes. Nor will the pressure be uniform. Tension also influences the voluntary action of muscles and can cause one's hands to tremble — a situation obviously to be avoided by a masseur.

A more subtle reason for the masseur or massueuse to be free from tension is that emotions are not confined to one's person — they are transmitted by mere proximity and by touch. There is a subtle exchange of feeling between the recipient and the masseur during a session. Emotion is transferable and known to be "contagious." Experiments have shown that even pets develop feelings reflecting those of the humans around them. And many experiments have proven that plants, too, respond to human emotions in very specific ways. It is clear then that if you are relaxed, it helps the other person to relax, and the massage will consequently be more productive.

The hands of the person receiving the massage should be kept apart, either on the arms of the chair or on his or her thighs. If the hands are clutched together, as is the habit of most people, energy currents sent from the head to the hands are shunted or short-circuited, and do not flow back to the organs. When one's hands are clasped, the two poles — the left, magnetic and negative, and the right, electric and positive — neutralize each other, thereby hindering the natural flow of magnetic current and electrical energy that courses up and down throughout the body.

Adjust the length of a session and the amount of pressure you bring to bear according to the recipient's reaction as indicated by facial expression.

Allow for short breaks between working on painful areas, so the pain is not continuous.

Work slowly and unhurriedly, giving the transmitted impulses the opportunity to more effectively clear blockages in the system.

The masseur's fingernails must be clipped closely — right down to the point of connection between the nail and the underlying tissue. Correctly trimmed, the thumbnail should appear to be one eighth of an inch shorter than the tip of the thumb. The nails themselves must be filed smooth, so they do not rub and sting the recipient's skin.

If you see that it is necessary, you may wish to give a brief explanation of the importance of correct posture, the right way of walking, good nutrition, and the proper care of the feet.

Explain also that the most beneficial results are obtained if the recipient can rest after a session, even nap if possible. Some of my clients have told me that they sleep deeply for an hour or more after a session. In any case, much activity is not advisable after a massage session. If the recipient has a long drive ahead, provide an easy chair so he may rest before starting. Any activity more intense than a short, slow walk home tends to diminish the results of even the best session.

Make the recipient aware that reflex compression massage is not a cure-all. Beneficial results do not depend exclusively upon receiving a good massage. One's attitude and subsequent behavior are also impor- tant. A massage is definitely helpful, but its benefits will be brief if the one receiving it continues to indulge in bad eating habits, and negative habits of thinking and living. Whatever good was done as a result of the massage will be effectively undone if negative patterns persist.

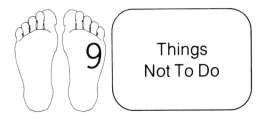

9 | Things Not To Do

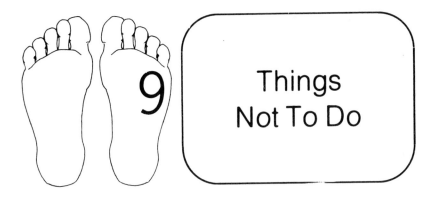

9 Things Not To Do

Do not use cream, lotion or oil on the recipient's feet, or your own hands. You must be able to feel the texture of the skin and discern whether the skin is dry or normal, as well as to discover which reflexes will require special attention. A person's skin gives a great deal of information concerning chronic problems and the level of tension in that individual.

Dry skin indicates a glandular imbalance in the thyroid, adrenals or the pancreas, and can indicate also that there is poor blood circulation. Tension causes the thyroid to be overworked and strained, consequently affecting the adrenal glands. If the skin is covered with oil, you have no way of discovering these things or the condition of the skin itself. Lotions will also cause the thumb to glide, making pinpoint accuracy on each point impossible. This results in missing some reflexes. And finally, if the thumb glides at all, the crushing of the crystalline deposits in the feet is not possible.

Do not press on either tendons or bones. Not only is it painful to do so, it is also useless for reaching subcutaneous reflex points.

Do not press on corns or thick callouses. Again, it is painful, and because this kind of tissue is not flexible, reaching subcutaneous points through them is impossible.

Do not press on injured places, varicose veins, swollen areas or scars. Pressure on any of these places may cause or increase injury, and these types of ailments heal very slowly, particularly in cases where poor circulation is involved. (Poor circulation is always associated with varicose veins and edema.) Causing any injury whatsoever is, of course, in direct conflict with the purpose of natural healing. If you are unable to work on the feet for any reason, work on the corresponding places on the hands instead. Stroke swollen feet gently from toes to knees, one leg at a time, using both hands.

Do not overdo it by either working too long at one session or by pressing too hard. Moderation in these two things is an absolute necessity. Eunice Stopfel's advice was that "it is better to undertreat than to overtreat." Overtreating, particularly in chronic conditions such as arthritis or diabetes, can result in a severe purificatory reaction within a day or two.

The recipient could feel really sick from the release of too many toxic substances into the blood. Never apply strong pressure if the recipient is diabetic. Reduce pressure right away if the slightest discoloration is noted, such as pinkish spots. This pink discoloration could become a bruise which might never heal. Particular care should be used if the recipient feels no sensitivity in an area that is normally sensitive. Numbness in the feet is often symptomatic of diabetes. The strength of pressure that you bring to bear also varies with every individual, so be sure to note how the recipient perceives it. If he thinks it is too heavy, diminish pressure accordingly.

During the session, keep conversation to an absolute minimum. Do not talk about anything not directly related to the present moment. Conversation about people or events puts the visual imagination to work, altering brain wave rhythms in the process. Thoughts are colored by emotions, which in turn influence brain waves, dividing the brain's reflex action. Vocal and mental stimuli activated by conversation, and the stimuli initiated by compression massage on the feet are conflicting and the massage is not as relaxing or effective as it should be. Conversation may also interfere with blood circulation, since thoughts and emotions cause vascular changes, dilating or contracting blood vessels and altering their normal rhythms of contraction and expansion. Ask the recipient to focus attention on the impressions and sensations felt as the massage progresses — you may get some interesting responses. One of my clients said, "I felt lightning going through me!" Another described a very pleasant wave of warmth flowing through her body. A writer told me that she could feel her brain "opening for new ideas." Still another said, "I see my problems evaporate — it is better than psychotherapy." It is worth noting that these people remained silent throughout their sessions.

Massage should not be given to anyone who has eaten a meal just before the session. The results would not be particularly beneficial, and nausea might even follow.

No person under heavy drug medication should be massaged. It could cause a purificatory reaction — a quick elimination of the drug from the system. The purposes and effects of medication and massage would, in this case, be in conflict with each other.

Do not massage anyone who has undergone recent internal surgery until the doctor has pronounced complete recovery.

Massage should not be administered to a pregnant woman unless (a) she has experienced it on prior occasions and felt relaxed after the previous massage, and (b) the pregnancy is a normal one, with no complications. Be very gentle, and keep the session brief.

Massage should not be given to a woman during menstruation. Excessive, prolonged bleeding, discomfort, and even some symptoms of poisoning could result. Nor should a masseuse give massages during her own menstrual period. Elimination is a function of the skin, and if some of the menopoison is on the hands of the masseuse, it will enter the pores of the recipient's skin, which obviously is not going to help that person feel any better.

Menstruation is a house-cleaning process: The female reproductive organs are meant to accept an embryo. If the ovum does not become fertilized, a reduction of the ovarian hormone progesterone occurs, and the mucous membrane and other tissues of the uterus rapidly disintegrate into a poisonous substance. Nature provides for its elimination through the menstrual flow. This is also one of the reasons why the menstrual blood does not coagulate — it has to flow out of the body. Experiments in Europe many years ago revealed that when rats were injected with extractions of the tissues and glandular fluid from menstrual blood, they died within ten minutes. Hence the name "menopoison." It was also well known in Europe that women in menstruation could not make bread — the dough did not rise because the yeast was apparently affected during kneading by the menopoison emitted through the skin. Massage speeds up the release of menopoison into the blood stream, and all organs are adversely affected by it.

Do not diagnose, prescribe, promise to cure, nor lead a recipient to believe that you can help a specific problem. To diagnose is to recognize and name a disease or ailment on the basis of symptoms. Only a licensed physician is legally permitted to diagnose. To prescribe is to offer advice or guidance for the purpose of aiding a condition recognized as a result of diagnosis. It implies to some degree the promise and hope of help. Again, only a licensed physician is permitted to prescribe. This whole area is extremely sensitive, subject to all kinds of interpretations, and it can be said that just about any kind of health advice borders on diagnosing or prescribing. Be very careful what and how you say things pertaining to the recipient's health.

For example, if you are told that a spot you just pressed was tender or painful, and you name the organ which corresponds to that pressure point, you are diagnosing, or suggesting that this organ may not be in good condition. If asked to identify the painful reflex and whether the organ is malfunctioning, your response might go something like this: "Because of the variety and complexity of body structures, the location of reflexes can only be approximated, and since I am not a doctor, I cannot tell you anyway." If asked why a particular point is sensitive, you can explain that because of the immense complexity of human physiology, there are many reasons for sensitivity. While we do want to be honest, we are not legally permitted to divulge a precise answer, even if we know it.

Should you be asked in person or by telephone if you can help someone with a backache, do not say yes, you can, because you really do not know if you can in the first place. Simply reply that you are not able to give a definite answer, but that reflex compression massage relaxes the entire body and relaxation has a beneficial effect on everyone and on all the body's functions. Explain further that you do not deal with, nor cure, ailments. You will be asked many times how long it will take for any particular condition to improve. But you must answer that neither the result nor the time necessary to improve can ever be accurately predicted. Even to advise a person as to which areas he or she could work on in order to improve a specific problem is prescribing.

Many want to know what reflex compression massage does to the system. You can truthfully reply that many aspects of reflexology are not yet completely understood or explained. Let them experience it and learn for themselves.

Never refer to your work as "reflexology." A massage license does not permit a claim that one is practicing reflexology. A reflex is a specific physiological change in an organ. Reflex massage causes physiological changes throughout the system, consequently, if you do not possess a medical license, you cannot say that you are doing reflexology. You can, however, call it relaxation massage, which will in no way diminish the value of your work.

Although these strict rules may be unreasonable, there is a positive side to it as well. To give a recipient anything resembling a diagnosis can incur unpleasant consequences. I recall a middle-aged woman and her fiancé, who were soon to be married, coming to me for a massage. While working on her feet, I found numerous sore spots corresponding to important organs. She kept asking me about the link between these sore spots and the organs of her body. Being eager to be of assistance and to teach her where and how she could work on her own feet, I told her that one of the sensitive spots reflexed to the liver, others to the kidney, the stomach, etc. A few days later she called to say that she felt much better after the massage, but that because of the distance she would not be in again. She also said she was reluctant to ask her fiancé to bring her because she did not want him to know about her ailments. He had shown a great deal of concern on the earlier visit, and she was worried that he might not marry her should he hear any more about her poor health. I promised to say nothing about her state of health at subsequent sessions, but still she decided against another appointment. The two were married. I learned later from mutual friends that she was constantly ailing and that there had been surgery because of the liver ailment. Here is a case in which my "diagnosing" at the initial session created harm. She was deprived of my further help because of it — help that could have changed things if the massage sessions had continued.

It is important to note that, as I learned firsthand, you can get into trouble with the law if you diagnose or prescribe. One time, a young man and a girl came to me. He complained of feeling tired and weak, and of having "weird heartbeats." He wanted a foot massage, and also asked that I instruct his girlfriend. I proceeded to do the massage and located some sore spots on his feet. I explained what that indicated, and told the young lady how and where to work. Then I showed them an herb book, in which I found an herb which regulates the action of the heart.

It was revealed later that the two were employed as undercover agents by the Consumer Protection section of the California Bureau of Food and Drug Administration. They had recorded the entire conversation with a hidden tape recorder. I was cited; and during a session with the Assistant District Attorney, I was told that by detailing to the young man matters concerning his health, I had violated certain legal codes. This, said the D.A.'s office, was diagnosing. And telling what to do about certain conditions was prescribing. I was warned not to do this in the future, and that if I continued, I might be arrested and charged with practicing medicine without a license. The session was most informative; I was grateful being able to receive legal information of which I had previously been unaware. Written as they are in legal terminology, the legal codes are often not perfectly clear. Interpretation is difficult, and only a professional prosecutor is in a position to evaluate any given situation. I share what I learned at that session with whomever is interested. It is my feeling that it is most important to be able to help people — you can do it as much as you wish, but be careful not to talk about it!

The First Amendment does, however, grant citizens the freedom of speech. I was told that this freedom extends to public lectures, seminars, classes, and writing articles or books. In a public lecture before a group of individuals, you are free to say whatever you believe or know about a subject. The Assistant District Attorney told me that one can even say, "Murder is good." The First Amendment allows this. In a seminar or workshop you may tell in detail what to do to solve specific health problems. But if you are a professional, and a client engages you for a massage and you are paid for it, the law *does not* permit you to tell what you found to be the problem, how to improve it, whether any improvement is possible, or how long it may take to improve the condition. Nor are you permitted to give dietetic counsel — this too is considered "prescribing." You may say, however, that "If I were in your situation, I would try this. . . ," or that some time ago you heard about a similar problem and that person did thus and so. You might then add, "You may try it if you wish." But make no definite statements. Helping others is a social and ethical obligation, but we must comply with the law even if it is unreasonable or "silly" as even the District Attorney admitted it is.

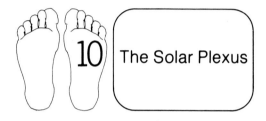

10 The Solar Plexus

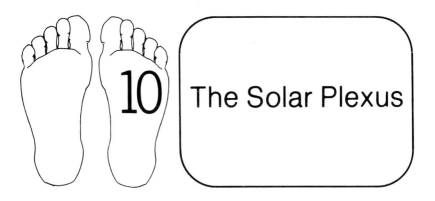

10 The Solar Plexus

The word "plexus" has its root in a Latin word that means "to braid." Anatomically, a nerve plexus indicates a network or a group of nerve fibers intertwined and very elaborately interlaced with each other.

The solar plexus is a very large nerve plexus located behind the stomach. *Taber's Cyclopedic Medical Dictionary,* (Appendix, page 57), calls it "the abdominal brain." The stomach is located in the left side of the body. The solar plexus is composed of two large ganglia from which many smaller ones in semi-lunar, or crescent shapes are distributed to many places.

There are about ten subdivisions. The ganglion is a mass of nerve tissue containing nerve cells. The ganglion is like a little energy center placed outside of the brain and spinal cord. Both of the solar plexus' ganglia are prevertebral, which means that they are located outside of the spinal column. One of them, called the celiac or abdominal, is located near the abdominal artery on the level where this artery originates. The other ganglion, which is the main one, is called "mesenteric," because it is connected to the mesentery, the fold of the membrane encircling the small intestines and forming a lining of the abdominal cavity. It is to be found on the *left side* of the abdominal aorta. This is the ganglion where the sympathetic nervous system originates, and from which the sympathetic fibers pass to the abdominal organs.

The sympathetic nervous system is therefore a part, a subdivision, of the solar plexus. According to its functions, the sympathetic nervous system is also a division of the part of the human nervous system which is called the autonomic nervous system; it controls and monitors the involuntary functions of human organs. These functions are performed automatically, and independently of our will — they cannot be consciously controlled. (There has, however, been recent evidence that some masterly adepts of the Yogic disciplines can consciously control certain of the "involuntary" functions.) These are the functions of glands and their secretions, the work of smooth muscles like the muscles of the internal organs, particularly the digestive tract, respiratory passages, walls of blood vessels and the heart, which supply energy for the assimilation of food.

The solar plexus, along with the sympathetic nervous system (which again, is a subdivision of the solar plexus), controls the marvelously orchestrated sequential events in our system, upon which our lives depend. The solar plexus presides over the sympathetic nervous system, and it is said that it is fully developed and already performing vital functions in the early stages of the human embryo — a time when even the brain is not yet developed. If the sympathetic nervous system is stimulated, as in a sudden upset, it works like an emergency station. It will cause the constriction of blood vessels, raise blood pressure, accelerate the heart, and allow a much greater expenditure of energy if that is necessary. It also inhibits the action of the intestines; thus prolonged tension will result in constipation.

The second division of our autonomic nervous system, the craniosacral part, is called the parasympathetic system. Stimulation of it increases the secretion of glands, lowers the blood pressure and slows down the heart.

Thus we see that the solar plexus is the greatest nerve center: It presides over most of the autonomic nervous system — it even organizes the blood circulation by changing the volume of blood that passes through the blood vessels; it regulates the circulation of vital forces and electromagnetic impulses flowing through the system.

Theron Dumont stated in his book, *The Solar Plexus,* that the solar plexus is also the source of vital force and physical energy and the great storehouse thereof, as well as being its generator. It actually has solar, sunlike qualities.

The solar plexus might be called also a "feeling brain." It is a center of feelings and emotions. One can experience a very special sensation in, and below, the chest when a strong emotion arises. People describe it as "getting sick to the stomach," but it is really a sensation in the solar plexus. The solar plexus sends messages or impulses through the nerves to corresponding organs, causing not only physiological changes, but also arousing particular mental states, which in turn influence one's physical condition. Every mental and emotional state has a physical manifestation. It is a well-known fact that an injury of the solar plexus disturbs the natural life processes, and a strong blow to this area can even cause instantaneous death.

The purpose of this detailed description of the location and function of the solar plexus is to emphasize that in order to obtain the best results in this work, it must begin on the left foot, and more particularly, from the solar plexus area, where the principal vital processes originate. Starting the reflex compression massage on this key area produces an initial relaxation in the solar plexus. This makes possible its natural functioning, which in turn causes the natural physiological responses of all the organs.

The solar plexus can be reached on both feet in spite of its location on the left side. The results of experience confirm it, even though there is no direct explanation as to why it is so. As the late Mrs. Eunice Stopfel has stated in her lectures, this is the only deviation from the straight zone pattern, in which the impulses elicited from the pressure points on the feet travel.

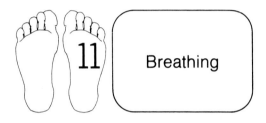

11 Breathing

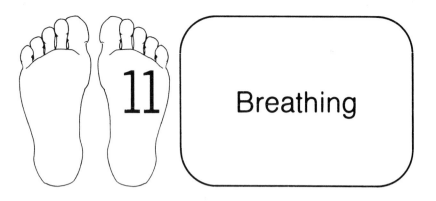

Breathing

Pay close attention to the breathing pattern of the recipient. It will provide valuable information for the work you do on the feet, and you will be able to give him or her some guidance in this respect.

Breathing performs many functions essential to life. It is one of the means of our communication with the external environment. Everything that exists must be, and is, in communication (in the broad sense) with the surrounding world.

There are two kinds of breathing: The automatic, unconscious breathing performed by all living organisms, and the conscious, controlled breathing we can choose to do for a specific purpose. It is good to know what is happening as we breathe. We can then be aware of some of the mechanics and functions of breathing when we breathe consciously.

During inspiration (inhalation), muscles raise the ribs and expand the chest cavity. One set of muscles acts on the ribs, another set acts between the ribs. The upper ribs are pulled upward by muscles extending from the neck down. Thus, breathing influences the condition of the neck, which is a place on the body that has much to do with whether one is relaxed or not. During expiration, the chest returns to its original size, and the muscles pull the ribs back down. The number of respirations under normal conditions ranges between 14 and 20 per minute.

Physiologically, breathing accomplishes two things: (1) The exchange of oxygen and carbon dioxide between the cells and their environment, a process which begins in the lungs and spreads from there, and (2) The consequent metabolic reaction of body cells and molecules to the incoming oxygen. It is a stimulus-response reflex action. Inhalation nourishes the system with incoming oxygen, distributed by the blood to every cell in the body; exhalation then removes carbon dioxide from the cells, as well as wastes and toxins, which completes the essential and necessary purification.

As it is a stimulus-response reflex action, breathing is intimately connected with the nervous system. Each is affected by the other. Breathing is directly related to blood circulation, heart rhythm, and not surprisingly, the skin condition.

Proper abdominal breathing influences and activates peristalsis, particularly on the small intestine. A progressive wavelike motion occuring involuntarily, peristalsis is very important in the functioning of the alimentary canal. This wavelike motion results in contraction and distension of the walls of the intestines, and in this way, their contents are moved on for eventual elimination. Thus, correct breathing even plays an important role in preventing constipation as well as other physical malfunctions.

Nervous tension partially blocks the flow of energy currents through the body, and even the most skilled reflexologist cannot remedy it fully. Your first step, then, is to observe the breathing pattern of the recipient when he is not thinking about it; that is, when the recipient is breathing as he or she normally does. Breathing has a definite psychological aspect — revealing as it does one's mental-emotional state. Shallow breathing indicates a person with a high level of tension; accelerated, short inhalations in a rapid tempo are evidence that one is emotionally upset, angry or fearful. Of course, pleasure too can cause increased heartbeat and rapid breathing. And pleasurable, interesting situations or scenes are said to be "breathtaking."

Almost instantaneous relaxation is induced by taking several deep, abdominal breaths. So suggest this to the recipient, adding that it should be done consciously and quietly. This exercise permits body cells to more effectively accept and utilize oxygen, improving the metabolic effect of breathing. By removing the blockage and permitting energy flow, this kind of breathing has a purifying effect, particularly in the nervous and lymphatic systems, facilitating improved coordination among all the organs, which is another prerequisite for health.

Quiet, controlled abdominal breathing produces a very pleasant feeling of freedom; it exerts an amazing influence on one's mental and emotional state. By all means, it is far more effective and decidedly preferable to tranquilizers. Abdominal breathing even induces a change in the pattern of brain waves, causing a shift toward the relaxed Alpha state. It balances, invigorates, and normalizes the system. And as Thomas Gaines states in his book *Vitalic Breathing,* (Concord Press, West Los Angeles, CA.), ". . .the act of breathing spreads the life-force through the body."

Pertinent facts about breathing and its relation to health should be concisely explained to the recipient. Those who become aware of its importance and discipline themselves to practice correct breathing, not only during a massage session but as part of a daily routine, will profit — and the results of your work will be more beneficial and of longer duration.

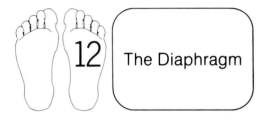

12 The Diaphragm

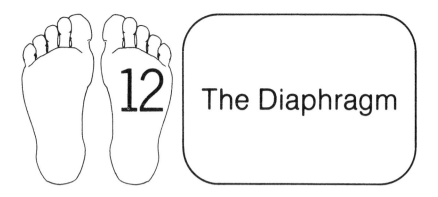

12 The Diaphragm

The diaphragm is a musculomembranous wall which separates the abdomen from the thoracic cavity. (Fig. 12) It contracts with each inhalation, flattening downward. This allows the lungs to descend and fill completely, all the way down to the lower part of the lung. The deeper the inhalation, the lower the diaphragm descends. This movement of the diaphragm presses the digestive organs down, which aids digestion and enhances the action of peristalisis of the intestines, pushing down food bulk by increasing intra-abdominal pressure until it reaches the stage of defecation.

With each exhalation, the diaphragm relaxes and rises, muscles pulling

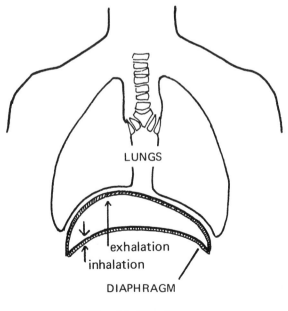

LUNGS

exhalation
inhalation

DIAPHRAGM

Fig. 12: Diaphragm

its "floor" upward. The more complete the exhalation, the higher it rises, but the right half always rises higher than the left. Thus, reaching the reflex to the diaphragm via the foot reflex point depends upon whether the recipient is inhaling or exhaling, and whether the right or left foot is being massaged.

All this points up the important role of the diaphragm. Proper elimination, of course, is essential to good health. Besides aiding in the eliminative process, the movement of the diaphragm appears to assist in the functioning of the adrenal glands, kidneys, liver, spleen, and the cardiac or upper end of the stomach by giving these organs a kind of gentle and rhythmic massage.

You will perform a service by advising people, particularly women, that tight girdles, belts, and tight-fitting figure adjusters interfere with the natural motion and function of these organs. If an individual has a particular problem with any of these organs, after the entire foot has been massaged, you may return for a moment to the reflex to that organ and to the diaphragm.

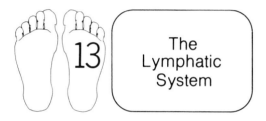

13

The Lymphatic System

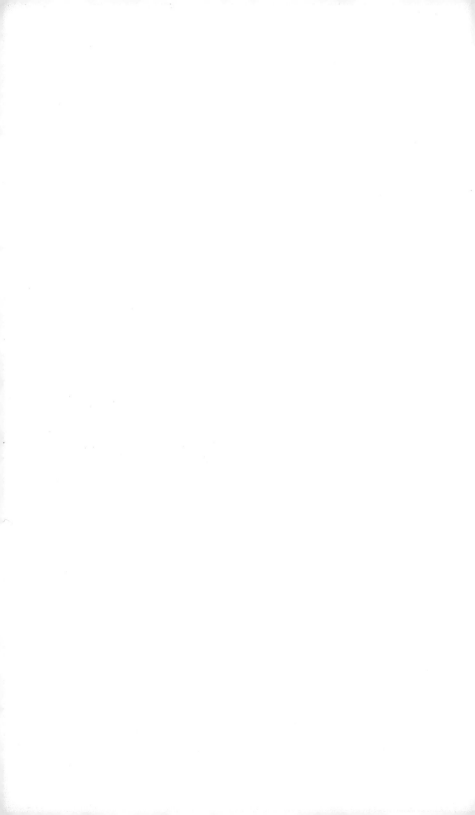

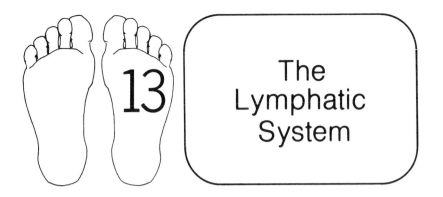

The Lymphatic System

The lymphatic system is part of the human circulatory system. Its function is essential for sustaining life. The system carries lymph from the body tissues to the points where it joins the blood stream. Lymph, the body's alkaline fluid, is formed in all of the body's tissues, gathered in the most minute blood vessels called capillaries, conveyed by them then to larger blood vessels, and finally, from there carried to the lymph ducts. Lymph is usually clear, transparent, and colorless, but it sometimes becomes milky when draining fats and wastes from the intestines. Its composition varies considerably in different parts of the body. Lymph contains cells called lymphocytes, which serve to protect the body against invading micro-organisms.

There are two kinds of structures in the lymphatic system: The first are the capillaries, the larger blood vessels and the lymph ducts, all of which serve to conduct the lymph through the system. Respiratory movements are also one of the important aids in the flow of lymph through the human body. There are valves in the lymph vessels which prevent any back flow of lymph. The second structures are the lymph nodes, functioning as a finely-tuned filter system.

The tissue fluid from the blood capillaries enters the lymph capillaries, and from this point is called lymph. There it is cleared and filtered from the waste products given up to it by the blood capillaries. It passes then through the larger lymph vessels and goes to the duct where it enters the blood stream. The tiny lymph capillaries lie in the connective tissue of most organs. They are most numerous under the skin, the mucous membranes of the respiratory and digestive tracts, and less numerous in the muscles.

Lymph vessels are much larger than the capillaries. Most of them lie in the subcutaneous layers of tissue, some are located deep in the extremities, as well as under the mucous membranes of the digestive, respiratory and urogenital systems. Unlike the blood, lymph flows in one direction only — from very small vessels to larger ones, and from there to lymph ducts, at which point it enters the blood stream. Lymph ducts are tubular channels through which the lymph flows to the veins.

There are two main ducts: The long thoracic duct on the left and the short lymph duct on the right. "Thoracic" indicates the lymph duct located in the chest. The thoracic duct is the principal one, conveying lymph from all parts of the body with the exception of the right side of the head, neck, upper chest and right upper extremity. The thoracic duct originates in the abdomen, and receives lymph from the lower limbs, the pelvic region and abdominal organs. It goes upward through the diaphragm into the thorax or chest, veers to the left and enters the vein under the left collarbone. Just before it enters this vein, the thoracic duct receives the flow of lymph from the vessels on the left side of the head, the left upper extremity and the left side of the chest.

The right lymphatic duct, the short one, is receiving the lymph only from the right side of the head, the right upper extremity and the right side of the chest. It empties into the vein under the right collarbone.

The thoracic duct is the larger of the two and is the main or principal one, serving a much larger area of the body and many more organs than the right lymphatic duct.

The other structures of the lymphatic system are the lymph nodes. These nodes are an accumulation of lymph tissues. They are rounded and densely packed with lymph tissue sacks. Lymph nodes vary in size from that of a pinhead to the size of an olive. They can occur singly or accumulate in groups in certain regions. The principal ones are in the neck, the armpits and the groin. They are both superficial and deep-seated. Their function is to act as a filter, so as to prevent bacteria and other harmful invaders from entering the blood stream.

Larger and more highly coordinated groups of lymph nodes appear in special forms that are termed "lymphatic organs." The lymphatic organs are the spleen, the thymus and the tonsils. The spleen, an elongated and ovid organ located on the left side of the body beneath the diaphragm and behind the stomach, is the largest lymphatic organ. It contains primarily a sponge-like substance consisting of lymphatic tissue. The major functions of the spleen are:

(a) The formation of blood cells and lymphocytes — white blood corpuscles.

(b) Blood storage.

(c) The filtration of foreign substances such as bacteria and worn out blood cells, which are destroyed and removed from the circulation by the action of the cells of the spleen.

(d) Storage of iron and saving it for the formation of new hemoglobin, a substance which carries oxygen to the tissues.

(e) The formation of antibodies and consequent immunogenic action. This function of the spleen plays a very important role in the resistance against bacterial and parasitic infections.

The thymus, the second of the lymphatic organs, is composed of very dense lymphoid tissue. It is located anterior to and above the heart; its primary function is to develop immunity in children. The last of the lymphatic organs are the tonsils. They too are filters against bacteria.

The lymphatic system is the most precious guardian against disease. In addition to the functions outlined above, the lymphatic system also regulates the amount of fluid in the vessels of the entire body and removes the proteins discarded by the blood capillaries. A malfunction in the system could cause edema and protein imbalance. The countless subdivisions of the lymphatic system work like a series of police stations, each subordinate to and dependent upon each other. Its master residences are in the left side of the body. And so, as the late Mrs. Eunice Stopfel often emphasized in her lectures, about 3/4ths of the body's toxins, being caught there by these "police stations," accumulate in the left side of the body. The body must be able to efficiently rid itself of these toxins. This is why it is so important that the lymphatic system have good drainage. An important prerequisite to good health is having an efficient circulatory system, a major part of which is a lymphatic system that is, to a high degree, free of toxins.

So it is that we find more reasons to start the reflexology session on the left foot. The pattern of alternating from the left foot to the right and back again can be found in Chapter 4. Additional reasons are given for starting work on the left foot in Chapter 10. If there are some particularly tender spots on the left foot, it is advisable to come back to them for a bit of brief, additional work.

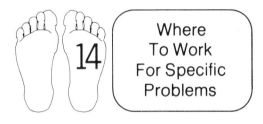

14 Where To Work For Specific Problems

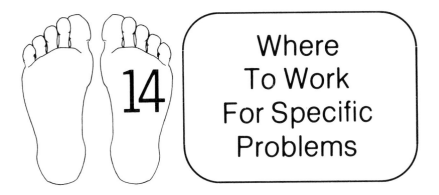

Where To Work For Specific Problems

14

Although the instructions in this chapter indicate where to work for specific problems, it is not implied that you must work only on these reflexes. Refer first to the chapter, *Things Not To Do*. Then massage the entire foot unless it is impossible or inadvisable to do so. Return to any specific problematic area and work briefly on them — you will find them to be less sensitive now. If it is not feasible to massage the whole foot, work on the specific areas if this is possible.

If a full massage is being given once or twice a week, you, or the recipient himself, may work on the specific areas listed here between sessions as often as several times a day if it seems advisable. When the work is done only on these specific reflexes, start by massaging the solar plexus reflex for a couple of minutes. As pointed out before, starting with the solar plexus relaxes the recipient before sore or sensitive spots are contacted and enhances the natural physiological responses of all the organs. A tingling or itching sensation felt during the massage indicates that circulation has been stimulated. Below is a brief outline of the specific reflexes to contact for particular ailments you may encounter.

Adrenal glands: Controlled by the sympathetic nervous system and responsible for hormone production, the adrenals regulate water distribution, are involved in muscle relaxation, resist fatigue, maintain a balance of minerals in the body and combat infections. A malfunction of the adrenals can cause excessive dryness of the skin and may contribute to allergies. If any of these disorders are manifest, work on the adrenals as well as on the ovaries and uterus, the testes, testicles and prostate gland, all of which have a functional connection to the adrenals.

Allergies: For hay fever and asthma, work on the organs indicated in the paragraph above and on the reflexes to the organs manifesting the symptoms — for aching or itching eyes, on the eye reflexes; for sore throat, on the throat reflexes.

Angina pectoris: Work on the reflexes to the solar plexus, heart, lungs, bronchial tubes, shoulders and the pituitary, adrenal and thyroid glands. A gentle, kneading massage directly on the shoulder muscles is also advisable.

Ankles: For swollen ankles, massage the reflexes to the heart and kidneys. Gently stroke the ankles upward, and work on the wrists, as the wrists and ankles are related.

Armpits: If there is some swelling or discomfort here, work on the fifth toes, their roots, the ball beneath the fifth toe and on the corresponding area on top of the foot.

Arthritis: Massage the reflexes to the particularly affected organs and areas, as well as the reflexes to the bronchial tubes, lungs, adrenals and the ileocecal valve. The ileocecal valve is a set of muscles that closes the passage between the small intestine and the ascending colon, preventing the re-entry of food material into the small intestine. Its malfunction causes excess mucus in the intestines, stomach and sinuses.

Asthma: First work on the reflexes to the solar plexus (again, for relaxation) since asthma is most often invoked by emotional stress. Then massage the reflexes to the bronchial tubes if they are in spasm, the lungs, adrenals and the thyroid. The thyroid is a pacemaker; it stimulates the adrenals, controls oxygen intake, and when this gland is overactive it causes nervousness and weight loss. If it is underactive, it causes overweight, dry skin, a sluggish mind, and raises the cholesterol level of the body. Examine the reflexes to the testicles, prostate, ovaries and uterus for tenderness or soreness. If they are so, work on them as well. The recipient may find it helpful to hold the tongue lightly with the teeth, without motion, for a few minutes several times a day.

Back: For stiffness and pain, reflex to the coccyx and the whole spine. I also recommend that you give the American Indian Massage.

Breasts: For swelling, cysts and lumps, work on the tops of the feet, the fifth through the second zones.

Breath: For shortness of breath work on the balls of the feet under the third and fourth toes.

Bursitis: Massage the top and bottom of the small toe, the outside edge of the foot, the reflexes to the shoulders under the small toe, the shoulder blades, upper cervical, the back of the neck and the kidneys. Reflex also to the hips because the hips and shoulders are related.

Calcium regulation: You need work only on the reflexes to the parathyroids.

Chest: For pain or discomfort in this area, massage the reflexes to the thoracic area of the spine, to the lungs, and on the top and bottom of the foot, fifth through second zones.

Cholesterol: For high cholesterol, reflex to the thyroid gland.

Common cold: Work on the reflexes to the affected areas such as the lungs and throat. For a head cold, be sure to work on the big toe. If the nose and sinuses are affected, massage the reflexes to the sinuses, which are on the balls of the fifth through second toes, returning briefly to the pituitary reflex. For acute colds accompanied by a high fever, work on the pituitary reflex every 15 minutes. If this is not possible, work on the thumb and fingers many times per day.

Constipation: The reflexes to the solar plexus, intestines and rectal area. To aid peristalsis, persons with this problem should do abdominal breathing every half hour or so for a couple of minutes. Repeat as well the following procedure several times a day: Press down on the center of the chin bone, just below the lower lip. *Do not* press on the gums or teeth. Maintain the pressure for a couple of minutes.

Diabetes: Work on the reflexes to the pancreas, pituitary gland, thyroid, adrenals, kidneys and the liver. Do all of these with extreme caution.

Digestive problems: The reflexes to the stomach, liver and colon. In addition, the recipient can firmly press the sides of his tongue with his teeth, first in a sort of kneading motion, then alternately press each side of the tongue, first the left, then the right, etc. The pressure should be held for just a moment and not too strong; be careful not to bite the tongue. This exercise greatly stimulates the flow of saliva, which of course aids in the process of digestion. It is worth noting that the digestion of all foods, except for meat, begins in the mouth. Also, if pressure is applied to the tongue just before putting food in the mouth, digestion will improve. It is said that the tongue possesses all the zones, so other organs will benefit from this exercise as well.

Emphysema: The reflexes to the bronchial tubes, lungs, sinuses, adrenals, the ileocecal valve, and the coccyx, which is often a very useful key to many problems.

Eustachian (auditory) tubes: Work on and under the root of the third toe, and on the joints of the third finger. For the ears and middle ears, work on the root and under the fourth toe, and on the joints of the fourth finger. Besides massaging the feet, work on the fingers at other times of the day, or on the fingers alone if you choose to work on yourself and are unable to reach your feet.

Eye: If the eye problem is mainly of a functional nature, massage the eye reflexes at the roots of the second and third toes. Work also on the pressure point on each foot in the center of the anterior edge of the shinbone, which is slightly above the area of reflexes to the glands in the groin.

Eye problems are associated with tension in the neck. Rotate the big toe for relaxation of the neck and work on the reflexes to the cervical area on the edge of the big toe. If glaucoma is involved, work also on the reflexes to the kidneys and intestines. If the eyes are crossing (Strabismus), work on the reflex to the coccyx. For cataracts, massage the parathyroids as well as the reflexes listed above. Herbalists tell us that tea brewed from celadine plants helps to dissolve cataracts, as does an extract of cineraria maritima applied with an eye dropper. The eyes and ears are closely related, so it is advisable to work on the reflexes to both. Some symptoms that could appear to be a cold, may not be. Watery eyes are related to a throat condition. Having a dryness and tickling sensation in the throat and a cough does not necessarily indicate that one has a cold. These symptoms could be pointing to a state of high tension, and relief may be pos-

113

sible by simply working gently on the jaws themselves and on the reflexes to the throat.

Fallopian tubes and the glands in the groin: Massage the tops of the feet, ankle to ankle.

Fatigue or weakened muscles: Work on the reflexes to the thyroid, parathyroid and adrenal glands. The adrenals regulate muscle tone.

Fever, fainting and unnatural skin pigmentation: Work on the reflexes to the pituitary and adrenal glands.

Gall bladder: Massage the reflexes to the liver and parathyroids.

Gas accumulation: Work on the reflexes to the ileocecal valve, the stomach and the sigmoid flexure, which is the lower part of the descending colon near the rectum.

Growth: If a child's growth is abnormally slow, you may be able to help by giving daily massage of the reflex to the pituitary gland, which secretes the growth hormone.

Headache: Headaches can be caused by many things — tension, eye strain, indigestion, earache, etc. Relief may be obtained by working on the big toes, particularly on their tips. Determine which are tender, then work accordingly — perhaps the reflexes to the colon, eyes, ears or the solar plexus. You can also work directly on the neck by pressing with three fingers of each hand about a half inch on each side of the spine's cervical portion.

Gentle pressure on each side of the nasal bone produces a relaxing effect which can sometimes be felt in the back of the head. This is one that can easily be done by the recipient himself. Another technique: Having the recipient press the roof of his mouth with a finger or the thumb often relieves a headache caused by eye strain or earache. Relief may result too, from a simultaneous, but not too strong pressure on both temples. This reduces excessive blood flow to the brain.

Heart: Massage the reflex to the heart on the left foot, the reflex to the shoulder blade; work on the fifth toe and on the seventh cervical. If the reflex to the colon is tender, massage it also. It is known that a heart disorder can result from the pressure pocket in the colon.

Hiccough: Work on the reflexes to the pituitary, solar plexus and the diaphragm. A hiccough is a spasmodic lowering of the diaphragm which causes periodic closing of the glottis. Hiccoughing can be elicited by blood pressure on the pituitary, irritation beneath the diaphragm, alcoholism, cerebral lesions, hysteria, disturbance of the phrenic nerve, or indigestion. If it is being caused by a temporarily overloaded stomach, massage must not be given at that time.

High blood pressure: First massage the reflex to the solar plexus. Then determine which reflexes are tender and attend to them. High blood pressure can have many causes, including colon toxicity and kidney trouble. If the kidney reflex is massaged, it is necessary to work also on the ureters and the bladder.

Hot flashes: Work first on the reflex to the pituitary gland, which regu-

114

lates the functions of all the glands in the body. Then work on the reflexes to the thyroid, ovaries and the neck.

Inflammation: Dr. Houston has indicated that inflammation anywhere in the body can be relieved by pressing the point on the soles of the feet, about two to two-and-a-half inches from the back edge of the heel (toward the toes), in the center of the foot at the junction of the arch and the ball of the heel.

Kidney stones: The reflexes to the kidneys, pituitary, thyroid and the parathyroids.

Legs: If the legs are puffy or swollen, drain the lymphatic system by "milking" between the big and second toes (see Chapter 3, Fig. 20). Massage the reflexes to the kidneys in order to increase urination, and work on the reflex to the adrenal glands.

Liver: Work on the reflexes to the liver and the thyroid, but do not do so more frequently than twice a week. Among its many other functions, the liver stores protein; it is also directly influenced by the thyroid gland.

Lungs: Massage all five zones, on the top and the bottom of each foot. Work also on the reflexes to the bronchial tubes (Area 10). Do the wrists and the tops of the hands as well.

Lymph glands: It is, of course, important to do the milking of the glands between the big and the second toe. To reach the lymph glands in the front of the body, particularly the breasts, massage the entire top of each foot. The lymph glands in the groin may be reached through reflexes on the top of the foot from ankle to ankle.

Mental sluggishness: Massage the reflexes to the pituitary and thyroid glands, and work on the tip of the big toe.

Migraine headaches: Work on the reflexes to the solar plexus, the tip of the big toe and the cervical reflexes on the edge of the big toe. Massage the reflex to the colon if it is tender, and work also on the reflex to the coccyx. The coccyx is the bone at the base of the spinal column which is composed of four fused rudimentary vertebrae. Once again, it is a key point to many areas and organs.

Mucus: In cases of excessive mucus, do the reflexes to the ileocecal valve and to the adrenals. A malfunction of the ileocecal valve is often caused by an insuffient cortisone supply from the adrenals.

Muscle cramps: Work on the reflex to the coccyx and on the parathyroids, which are the body's calcium distributors. Muscle cramps are often caused by a lack of calcium in the muscle.

Neck: Tension and stiffness in the neck are often the result of impaired drainage of the lymphatic system, and so tension spreads to the shoulders. Work on the drainage by milking the lymphatic system. Massage the points on the vertical line nearest the second toe between the top and root of the big toe, and the root of the big toe itself. Also do the reflexes to the cervical area of the spine and those to the shoulder area. Gently rotate, or "circumduct," the big toe. You should also press directly beneath and above the collar bone.

Nervousness: Massage the reflexes to the solar plexus, and the pituitary and thyroid glands. For relaxation, you can massage these reflexes daily.

Sciatica: For pain along the sciatic nerve, start the massage from the outside edge of the left foot at a point about two-and-a-half to three inches from the heel and proceed down to about one inch from the heel. Return to the starting point and work across the foot to the spinal line at the inside edge of the foot. This is the lumbar area. At this point, change the angle and work on the spine toward the heel as far as you wish. Then massage the outside top of the foot, starting about one-and-a-half inches from the heel on the outside edge, and proceed toward the ankle bone. Press the reflexes to the hip, then move along the Achilles tendon to about two inches above the ankle. Repeat this procedure on the right foot. Work also on the reflexes to the kidneys and bladder because uric acid usually is one cause of sciatica. The colon can cause it also, so work on this reflex, as well as on the prostate gland which, if enlarged, contributes to the irritation of the sciatic nerve.

The sciatic nerve, the largest nerve in the body, starts from the sacral area and extends down to the back of the thigh, dividing there into two parts, one extending along the tibia (the inner larger bone of the leg), down to the ankle. The other part of the sciatic nerve extends along the fibula, the thin outer bone between the knee and ankle. This explains why we find reflexes to the sciatic nerve in so many places.

Shoulder Joint: Rotate the fifth toe and work on the ball beneath it. An injury to the shoulder could even affect the lumbar area, so work on that reflex, as well as on the reflexes to the shoulder blade and the neck.

Skin: If the skin is dry, discolored by a yellowish pigmentation, or if there are skin eruptions, massage the reflexes to the liver, pituitary, thyroid and the adrenals.

Sinuses: Massage the big toe and the balls of all the other toes. Do the reflex to the ileocecal valve. And if the recipient's digestion is faulty, massage the reflexes to the intestines.

It is also helpful for the sinuses to spray a mixture of one part lemon juice to three parts warm water into the nostrils twice daily. Bathing the eyes in lemon juice diluted with water in the morning and in the evening may also be helpful. Lemon possesses disinfectant qualities.

Small Intestines: Massage all five zones on each foot.

Varicose veins: Massage the reflexes to the adrenals and the parathyroids. As noted above, the adrenals regulate muscle tone. If digestion is a problem, work on the reflexes to the intestines, and on the forearms and elbows on the places that directly correspond to the affected areas on the legs. You will have to estimate the zones. Phlebitis and varicose ulcers result from both impaired circulation and (quite often) a malfunction of the colon.

Vocal cords: To strengthen the vocal cords, massage the big toe and the portion nearest the second toe. Do also the reflexes to the throat. The recipient himself can massage the sides of his nose.

Water retention: To help relieve puffiness in the extremities, massage the reflexes to the adrenals, heart and the kidneys.

Weight: If either underweight or overweight, massage the reflex to the thyroid. If there is constipation as well, work on the reflexes to the intestines.

Whiplash: Massage the reflex to the cervical area, which is on the edge of the big toe. Work on the ball of the foot, below both the big and second toe; also on the reflexes to the neck and shoulders, and rotate the big toe.

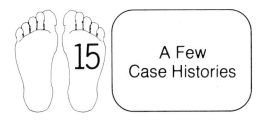

15

A Few
Case Histories

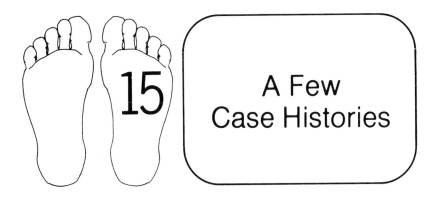

15

A Few
Case Histories

It may be useful to examine several case histories that I have encountered. You will find that there are no "typical" cases. All cases that you take on require your full attention and care. And, as pointed out earlier (in Chapter 8), the masseur has a responsibility to the recipient to be as free as possible from tension and negative emotion. This is because there is a subtle exchange of feeling between the recipient and the masseur during the session. Positive and lasting results are not the result of a mere mechanical employment of the techniques. The more relaxed and clear you are about the service you perform for others, the more the session will benefit the whole person.

A man in his mid-twenties, looking thin, weak and tired, came to me for a massage. He told me that he had lost his appetite and that he was losing weight even though he was forcing himself to eat. No one had as yet been able to learn what was wrong. Following a few sessions of compression massage however, this young man was eating normally again, had noticeably more energy, and was gaining weight and strength.

Pain, stiffness of the neck and a constantly stuffed nose were the complaints of a man who said he had had the neck condition for about a year. He was not able to move his head from side to side at all, and the severely blocked nasal passages were apparent the moment he began to speak. But after a few sessions he could move his head, and his nose had cleared. "You're a healer!" he exclaimed. The "healer," I explained, is the ancient method of the body healing itself based upon a deep wisdom and knowledge of the nature of the human system.

Red spots covering the face of a woman who came to me were caused, she said, by "some kind of allergy." There was a constant itching, and she just could not keep her hands away from her face. After 20 minutes of massage the itching ceased, and after a few more sessions, it stopped altogether. I then taught her how and where to work on her feet, and instructed her to do so daily, so that she no longer required my services.

A woman in her 50's who had advanced cancer in the left breast came to me once a week for massage. Her entire left arm and hand were so swollen that they looked shapeless, and she could hardly bend the arm.

The swelling diminished markedly after each session, remaining that way for three days, during which she felt much better. But in this case, unfortunately, the improvement could not be permanent.

A certain young man kept making appointments for massage even when it seemed he did not really need them. He was healthy, but his feet were tender. After several sessions the tenderness was not nearly as pronounced, but he kept coming. I finally asked why he continued to return. He then told me that the session served as a form of psychotherapy for him: He felt relaxed for a week following each session, slept well for the first time in years, handled his problems and job with more skill, and even his memory had improved. "You have magic hands," he said.

A young woman came to me with a lump the size of a walnut in her armpit. She had been scheduled for surgery. She came to me for several sessions, after which the lump disappeared. She informed me that when she first came, she did not really believe that the problem could be helped through massage, but she had wanted to try a form of natural healing before going in for surgery. How fortunate that she did!

I often hear people make comments about their own experience with reflexology which are quite similar to the experiences of many others as well. One comment frequently heard is that after the session the recipient feels as if he or she is "walking on air," or that they feel "weightless, just like a feather." They speak of the "wave of warmth" flowing through the body, the sensation of "lightning" passing through them, or of feeling that they are "opened up" to new ideas or sensations.

Sometimes however, the results are not so spectacular. A woman in her early forties came to see if I could help her. She had suffered from rheumatoid arthritis from early childhood, was in constant pain and received cortisone injections regularly. I was extremely cautious, and worked gently on the reflexes to the solar plexus and on the big toe of each foot as well for about five minutes only. She called me later to tell me that she had been so sick the evening after receiving the massage that she could not report for work on the following day. This was, of course, a powerful purificatory reaction of her system. She returned a week later, and we both hoped that the reaction would gradually lessen in intensity. We tried it for five weeks, with no easing of the severe reactions whatsoever. Evidently, after 35 years of this chronic condition, her body had become so saturated with toxins and medication that the purification process would take a very long time. Eventually she would have been helped, but who can say how much? Since she could not afford to miss one work day a week, we decided — to our mutual regret — to forego further sessions.

A woman in her early thirties came to me crying. When I asked her what the problem was, she replied that she was perfectly healthy and she did not know exactly why she had come. But a brief interview revealed that she was upset because she was about to lose her secretarial job. She had been making so many mistakes that her boss informed her that unless she improved she would soon be fired. I was happy to learn that after a few sessions her concentration and the speed of her work had improved a great deal — to the point where she made almost no mistakes. Her boss praised her performance and even gave her a raise in salary. "You saved my job!" she said.

Another woman, weak, nervous, and afflicted with pains in the joints throughout the body, found relief for two days after the massage session, after which the pain returned. I then learned from her husband that she virtually lived on coffee and doughnuts. She drank 20 cups of coffee a day, and had doughnuts as often as five times a day! He found it necessary to cook for himself in order to get more nutritious food. My time and effort had been wasted, since she refused to change her eating habits — which actually stemmed from a mental-emotional condition. I had to stop giving her massage.

So be prepared: Some cases, for whatever reason, cannot be helped. I am not sure of the percentage of such cases, but Eunice Stopfel said that about 20 percent of the cases one encounters do not respond either partially or completely. Do not expect miracles, though some do happen. And when there are instances that compression massage does not help, do not be discouraged.

Sometimes during the session there is an instant reaction: The feet and hands perspire so that they are practically wet and the person says that the whole body perspires. It is a purificatory response of the glands.

In one case a woman who came had severe bursitis and also marital problems — she was almost on the verge of divorce. After a few sessions her bursitis was gone and because she became calmer and more open-minded her marital problems disappeared. She told me "You saved my marriage — I wish I could take you home with me — it would make the whole family happy."

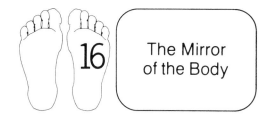

16

The Mirror
of the Body

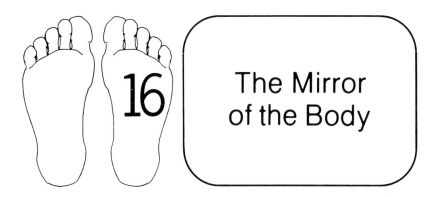

The Mirror
of the Body

The feet really amount to being the mirror of the body. So stated Robert Samilson, M.D., former president of the American Orthopedic Foot Society, in the October 1973 issue of *Today's Health* magazine. The feet are miraculous structural masterpieces, exquisitely and beautifully designed, a perfect coordination of many muscles — extrinsic, intrinsic, elastic, tissue, ligaments, capsules and more. Comprised of 26 bones, 100 ligaments, 20 muscles, and an intricate network of nerves and blood vessels, these marvelous structures also reflect totally our state of health.

The condition of our feet, and the way we use them, reveals our physical and mental state, and influences not only their own performance but the functioning of our mind and body as well. How we think and act has a direct bearing on how our feet do their job. Likewise, how we treat our feet influences our mental and physical health. It is a two-way street, a reciprocal relationship: Abusing the feet and the consequent foot ailments like blisters, bunions, callouses and corns often causes in turn general fatigue and bodily aches.

Conversely, systemic or general body disorders such as rheumatoid arthritis, diabetes, multiple sclerosis, and some types of heart diseases show up first in the feet, causing them to hurt some time before the malfunctioning organs have exhibited other symptoms. Foot pain can indeed camouflage serious diseases, so foot discomfort of any kind demands immediate attention — not only to the foot, but to the rest of the body. What may appear to be merely a foot problem could in fact be a symptom of a systemic disease.

Medical statistics reveal that three out of four Americans are plagued with one or more foot problems. Let's look at some of them:

Athlete's foot, while not a disease in itself, represents an entire set of symptoms — scaling between the toes, an itching sensation and a softening of the flesh are the most common of the symptoms. It may initially be the result of a fungus, but if it becomes chronic, roughening of the skin can follow. Known technically as hyperkeratomycosis, which is the thickening and hardening of the external layer of the skin, athlete's foot occurs more frequently in men than in women. It may be a local problem, but it can also be a result of an allergy, a drug overdose or a sunburn. I once saw a case where it had been caused by an overdose of Vitamin D.

Bunions are another foot problem. The predisposition to bunions might be inherited, but we know too that a bunion can develop from poorly fitted shoes. In some, but not in all cases, the "bursa" or sack over the joint of the big toe becomes inflamed and swollen, sometimes twisting the big toe under the next one. When working on a person with such a condition and for whom it is painful, you must work on the corresponding place on the hand. Pressure must not be applied to swollen areas.

It is estimated that 8 million Americans suffer from corns and callouses. They can be a result of friction, abnormal foot structure, systemic problems, or even of glandular imbalance and mental or emotional upsets. In Chapter 6 we described how a 28-year-old woman developed thick callouses within a matter of days while undergoing extreme stress after learning that her husband had left her. That was a dramatic demonstration of how the emotions profoundly influence the body and the feet in particular. A chiropodist or podiatrist will usually prescribe salicylic acid plasters to remove corns and callouses. Castor oil rubbed twice daily into the affected area softens the corn or callous so that it can eventually be peeled off with the fingers. Other home remedies one might use are the application of a thin slice of lemon fastened with a band aid or adhesive tape and left for the night; or one could apply a piece of cotton dipped in witch hazel to the area for the night. After a number of applications over a period of several days, the skin usually softens enough to gradually remove the corns and callouses.

Many people are born with a predisposition to fallen arches, but may never suffer from it. While arch supports may be helpful in certain circumstances, specifically designed exercises are preferable. It is interesting to note that through the centuries, superstitions or myths have developed about the arches of the feet. One such myth is that high arches are a sign of aristocratic descent. Low arches may be an ethnic characteristic, and yet cause no pain. Most blacks have flat feet, but almost never have the foot pain associated with them. Millions of people have exceptionally low or "flat" arches, but have had no pain or foot problems. The condition is not necessarily abnormal, and whether one's arch is high or low is not of prime importance. It is true that arches are important for healthy feet and posture, but the flat foot is not always a troublemaker, by any means.

Morton's Neuroma is another problem which can become acutely painful. It is characterized by a thickening around the nerve in the ball of the foot, and it is so painful that the ball of the foot can hardly be touched. A numbness between the toes frequently accompanies this disorder, which is sometimes marked by sensations of pain that shoot up from the toes like an electric shock. Relief might be obtained by soaking the feet in an epsom salt solution, or bathing with Dr. Scholl's foot soap. A transverse arch support also might be helpful. The person suffering from this ailment often finds it necessary to wear wide shoes. Local foot troubles often result from ill-fitting shoes, neglect, incorrect walking habits, incorrect posture while standing for extended periods, or even faulty eating habits.

One thing is certain: All foot problems and abnormalities *affect the entire body.*

Feet symptoms of systemic diseases:

Rheumatoid arthritis in its early stages may appear as pain, stiffness, or swelling in the joints of the feet. Tiny lumps beneath the skin, known as subcutaneous nodules, may appear as early warning signs of this serious ailment. You can feel these nodules very distinctly under your thumb or fingers. Press gently because you may release too much toxin at one time for the recipient to handle comfortably. When the disease has reached the degenerative, chronic stage, deformities such as hammertoes and bone spurs may appear.

Appearing more frequently in men than in women, gout is one of the common forms of arthritis. It is possible to be genetically predisposed to arthritic ailments. Even though people who are so disposed have a so-called "arthritic factor" in their blood, it does not mean that it has to develop. Its appearance is often marked by a sudden change in the big toe, which becomes shiny, swollen, inflamed, and extremely painful. The initial point of irritation is usually the junction of the big toe and the ball of the foot, but other joints in the feet may also be affected. While at first perhaps mistakenly viewed as a local problem, eventually gout comes to be known for what it is.

Gout is caused by a disturbance in the uric acid metabolism, which results in a buildup of water in the body. Because of an excess of waste products in the system, insoluble uric acid salts accumulate in the blood around the joints, and in the tissue itself in the form of crystalline deposits which one can feel when they are pressed. Medical authorities indicate that being merely 10 percent overweight is enough to trigger a preexisting asymptomatic condition. Thus, individuals who watch their weight and get adequate exercise are less apt to develop gout.

Cardiovascular diseases — those affecting the heart and circulatory system — may cause pain, swelling, and a burning sensation in the feet if blood circulation is impaired.

Arteriosclerosis, which is the hardening and thickening of the arteries, seriously reduces blood flow, with a consequent loss of oxygen to the tissues of the feet. Difficulty in walking, pain when the feet are at rest, ulcers, infections, loss of hair on the legs, and the thickening of the nails — particularly on the big toes — are all clues to the presence of this disorder.

Swelling and edema in the feet and legs can be caused by heart inadequacy. Body fluids then accumulate in the extremities, since they are restricted in their flow.

An early symptom of diabetes is often a numbness and a tingling sensation in the feet. Ulcers may develop on the soles, and if infections occur, they heal very slowly.

Symptoms of neurological problems or nerve disorders, even brain lesions, can appear in the feet in the form of lack of coordination. Alcoholism causes numbness and ulceration on the feet from nerve degeneration. A loss of muscular coordination, tingling and trembling, numbness, and difficulty in maintaining one's balance may be signs of multiple sclerosis.

Observing symptoms and knowing what they may indicate provides you with valuable information as to which organs may be affected, alerting you to the corresponding areas requiring special attention.

If you give your feet the kind of care they deserve, the entire system will benefit, and one's mental ease and general good health will be easier to achieve.

Here are some tips on proper care of the feet:

Insist on wearing shoes about a half inch longer than your foot.

Buy shoes in the afternoon — one's feet expand during the day. Leather shoes or fitted sandals are best. If you wear socks, they should be wool or cotton, and about a half inch longer than your feet.

If possible, change shoes twice a day.

After bathing, dry the feet carefully between the toes, then rub gently with an *edible* oil.

Stimulate foot circulation by alternately soaking the feet in warm and cool water.

While lying down, place a pillow under the feet to elevate them slightly.

Do not cross your legs while sitting because it hinders blood circulation and affects the spinal nerves.

It is best not to wear garters, hose or socks because all of these items of apparel impair circulation.

Walk as much and as often as you are able for relaxation and exercise.

Used correctly and naturally, our feet can be healthy and provide the body with good service. Consequently, it can be very useful to us to know their function. Two important jobs the feet perform are supporting and maintaining one's posture and propelling the body in whatever direction we desire. Both walking and running are affected by one's gait and the degree of dexterity we have in performing these basic functions. If these two characteristics of movement — gait and dexterity — are in line, then normal feet will be comfortable under most conditions. It is estimated that the force to which each foot is subjected during a single day is equivalent to approximately 600 tons for a 150-pound person. All movement involves the neuromuscular mechanism, and the necessity of nourishment by the vascular and lymphatic systems. The talus, or ankle bone, is the key to the normal functioning of the feet. As John McMennel, M.D., states in *Foot Pain* (Little, Brown & Co.), the talus is "a very unique bone." There are no muscles attached to it, and if its movement is impaired or habitually incorrect, pain in the foot will result.

One's posture and gait are individual characteristics, but they depend upon the work of the feet. Faulty posture stretches and tightens the ligaments, causing pain in the feet. If one's work requires long periods of standing, the feet should be kept at *hip width* to help maintain the lateral balance of the trunk. Standing motionless for extended periods can cause pain and should be avoided. If there are problems in any of the areas of posture, gait and coordination of the feet, retraining in this respect can be very useful and important.

When standing, the feet should be parallel. If angled outward, the hip muscles contract, causing strain on the ligaments and consequent discomfort. (Fig. 13) So, keep the shoulders back and down. They should be relaxed and not held stiffly. One's head should be straight up, "as tall as possible," with the neck relaxed and the chin in. The chin should not be extended forward because this position adversely affects the proper vertical flow of gravitational force through the body. One's pelvis should be "rolled under" when standing. The sacrum, a triangular bone forming the posterior section of the pelvis, supports the vertebral column and serves the articulation of the legs. The "gravity line" extends through the sacrum, and is balanced there with the energy of the individual, insofar as it is a center of polarity, the sacrum influences the position of the spinal column, and is the center of many reflexes. In addition to this, the structural condition of the sacrum and its position influences the skin and mucus distribution in the system.

Correct pelvic posture decreases the stress of weight on the feet. Incorrect posture can cause irritation of the spinal nerves, resulting in pain along the back to the head, arms, forearms, abdomen and chest, down to the front of the thighs, calves, and into the lateral parts of the feet and heels. The misuse of body energy in this way depletes its supply, which manifests in fatigue and lowered vitality. (Fig. 14)

The correct walking gait should be done with the feet nearly parallel and the toes slightly pointed out. One's soles should be flat on the floor, not tilted sideways, which puts weight unequally to one side. When the heel contacts the surface, the foot begins its propulsive function. This should occur along the central line of the foot, with a gentle rotating movement of the hips — otherwise a strain is placed on the ankles, the toes may be improperly positioned, and a deformity can result.

So observe how the recipient walks. If there is a complaint about pain in a specific area, in the heels for example, you must be aware that the organ corresponding to the heels *might not* be the culprit. You should pay special attention to the spinal reflexes, and give the person some valuable instruction on the proper way to walk and stand.

It is usually assumed that when standing barefoot, the body's weight is evenly distributed. But biomechanic researchers in the Cleveland Clinic Foundation learned that even in persons with normal feet, weight distribution between the heel and the ball of the foot is not equally balanced. They found that weight distribution is almost never ideally balanced, with variation usually ranging between 40 percent and 60 percent. Unequal distribution of weight makes one uncomfortable and causes fatigue. There are corrective exercises, but they may be different for each individual. Proper shoes are also necessary. To attain equal weight distribution,

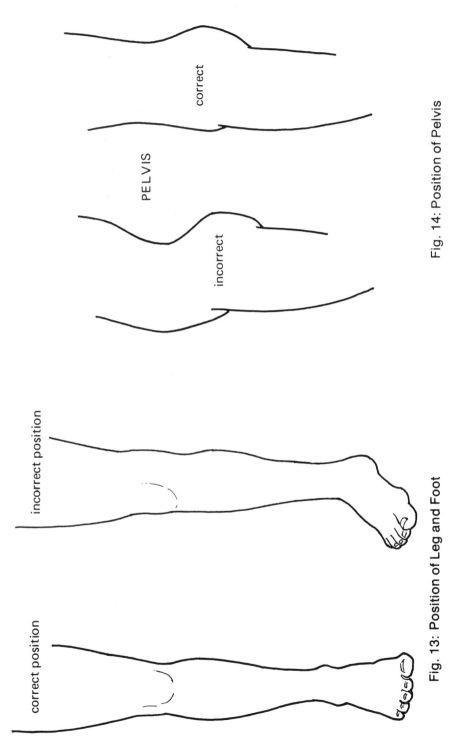

Fig. 14: Position of Pelvis

PELVIS

correct

incorrect

incorrect position

correct position

Fig. 13: Position of Leg and Foot

132

some may require shoes with the "negative heel," as in the Earth Shoes, while others may need higher heels or even wedge-type heels.

Dr. Yaichiro Hirasawa, professor and researcher at Shizuoka University in Japan, has confirmed the almost uncanny relationship between our feet and the rest of the body. Dr. Hirasawa has invented a "pedoscope" which, when an individual stands on the machine, makes a print indicating where the center of gravity is in that person's body. If the center is "off," it indicates that there may be trouble in corresponding areas. Exercises are then used to correct the posture. The special exercises and programs he has developed are used in centers for retarded children in Canada, Mexico and the United States. According to an article in the *National Enquirer* (Oct. 7, 1974), the method is being explored and used in the Texas Medical Center, Houston, by Dr. Makoto Igarashi, director of the center's College of Medicine. Dr. Igarashi sees the pedoscope as "an important development."

The article goes on to point out that Dr. Hirasawa reports a 90 percent rate of success using foot characteristics as a diagnostic tool. The study of some 75,000 patients reveals that the toes are particularly helpful as a guide in detecting illnesses and disease. He has found, for example, that a painful and stiff big toe usually signifies liver trouble, and pain or stiffness in the second and third toes reveals the presence of a stomach problem. Pain and stiffness in the fourth toe, he says, is related to a spleen condition, while pain in the little toe suggests a bladder problem. If one of the toes does not make full contact with the surface, it can indicate digestive or respiratory trouble. If all the small toes are considerably shorter than the big toe, there may be a problem with emotional instability. And finally, slippers which inhibit the use of the heels can cause headaches.

As we consider the vital relationship of the feet to the well-being of the body, we are reminded of the observation of Dr. D.D. Palmer, founder of the science of chiropractic: "The action of the body and organs," he said, "is highly intelligent." Dr. Palmer believed that an "Innate Intelligence, the inner mind," controls the body mechanism through the brain and nervous system. Interestingly, the ancient Greek physicians spoke also of the inner intelligence, some believing it to be a part of the Universal Intelligence. The highly respected philosopher Teilhard de Chardin tells us that "every cell in the human body contains part of the Cosmic Intelligence."

The feet contain this same intelligence. And since they play such a crucial role in the healthy functioning of the human system, assuredly they deserve as much "Tender Loving Care" as we can give them.

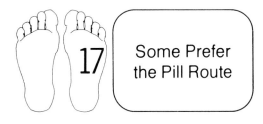

17　Some Prefer
the Pill Route

17 Some Prefer the Pill Route

The approach we have been considering is a holistic one, that is, one that views health in terms of the whole person, and sees the body as an integrated organism of many parts and nuances, each of which must function correctly if the others are to do their job. This holistic approach has brought relief across a wide spectrum of conditions. Indeed, success is limited virtually only in the cases of those with a chronic ailment, and then not because the condition cannot be helped, but because the reactions may be so severe over an undetermined period of time that it may well interfere with work. And of course one cannot help people who, because of temporary discomfort or inconvenience are unwilling, or because of economics, unable to spend the time required for recovery.

Everyone who experiences reflex compression massage can benefit from it, but not all will recover completely. No matter what may be done in terms of massage and counsel, some will continue to eat the wrong foods, drink the wrong beverages, and refuse to give up smoking, drinking or taking drugs. These people refuse to alter their mental attitudes about themselves and the world, and so they cannot be helped.

We who administer this form of massage are not doctors. We refuse to "cure" any person or condition, or to promise a cure. We do not diagnose or prescribe. We apply specific techniques to induce relaxation and to restore proper circulation and polarity balance.

But why is reflexology not more widely used, since it is not at all difficult to master the technique? Probably it is because such methods are considered to be just too much work. Our culture has developed an "instant remedy" psychology — a pill for this, a pill for that. Too often we find it easier to go the apparently easy route: Let the doctor fix me up.

Location
of
Reflexes

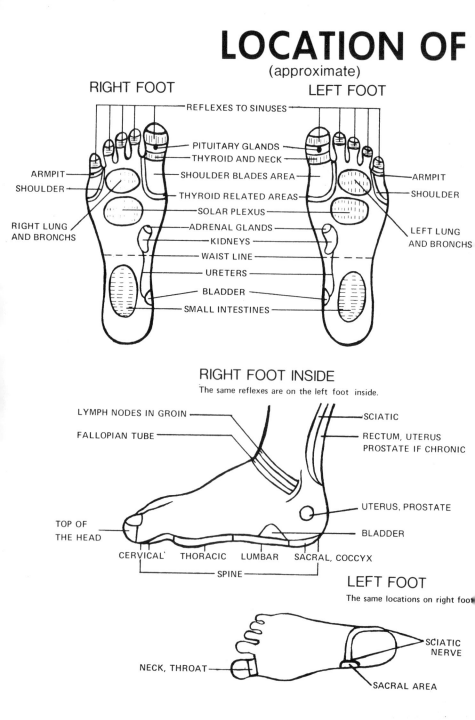

LOCATION OF
(approximate)

RIGHT FOOT   LEFT FOOT

REFLEXES TO SINUSES

PITUITARY GLANDS
THYROID AND NECK
ARMPIT   SHOULDER BLADES AREA   ARMPIT
SHOULDER   SHOULDER
THYROID RELATED AREAS
SOLAR PLEXUS
RIGHT LUNG   ADRENAL GLANDS   LEFT LUNG
AND BRONCHS   KIDNEYS   AND BRONCHS
WAIST LINE
URETERS
BLADDER
SMALL INTESTINES

RIGHT FOOT INSIDE
The same reflexes are on the left foot inside.

LYMPH NODES IN GROIN   SCIATIC

FALLOPIAN TUBE   RECTUM, UTERUS
PROSTATE IF CHRONIC

UTERUS, PROSTATE

TOP OF   BLADDER
THE HEAD
CERVICAL   THORACIC   LUMBAR   SACRAL, COCCYX
SPINE

LEFT FOOT
The same locations on right foot

SCIATIC
NERVE
NECK, THROAT

SACRAL AREA

Fig. 15: Approximate Location of Reflexes

REFLEXES

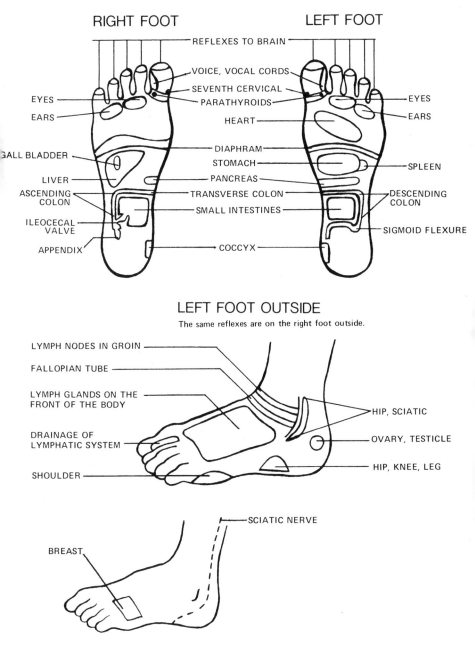

RIGHT FOOT   LEFT FOOT

REFLEXES TO BRAIN

VOICE, VOCAL CORDS

SEVENTH CERVICAL

EYES   PARATHYROIDS   EYES

EARS   HEART   EARS

DIAPHRAM

GALL BLADDER   STOMACH   SPLEEN

LIVER   PANCREAS

ASCENDING COLON   TRANSVERSE COLON   DESCENDING COLON

SMALL INTESTINES

ILEOCECAL VALVE   SIGMOID FLEXURE

APPENDIX   COCCYX

LEFT FOOT OUTSIDE

The same reflexes are on the right foot outside.

LYMPH NODES IN GROIN

FALLOPIAN TUBE

LYMPH GLANDS ON THE FRONT OF THE BODY

HIP, SCIATIC

DRAINAGE OF LYMPHATIC SYSTEM

OVARY, TESTICLE

SHOULDER   HIP, KNEE, LEG

SCIATIC NERVE

BREAST

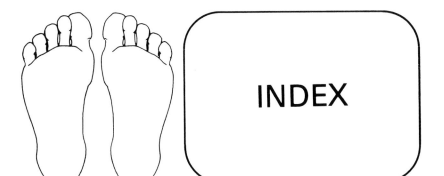

INDEX

neurological problems, 129
neurons, 12
  afferent, 12, 13
  efferent, 12, 13
New Mind, New Body, 69

oil, use of in massage, 85
ovary, 50, 52, 111
overweight, 112, 117

Palmer, Dr D, 133
pancreas, 45, 85
parasympathetic system, 94
peristalsis, 98, 101, 113
pituitary gland, 76
polarity, 17
  reflexes, 17
Polarity Therapy, 17
position of the feet, during
massage, 31
  masseur, 29
  recipient, 29
pregnancy, 86
pressure, 69-72
  of the thumb, 25
  points, 25, 26
prostate, 49, 50, 111
  enlarged, 116
protoplasm, 13
The Puzzle of Pain, 71

receptors, 71
rectum, 48, 49
reflex, 23
  allied, 14
  antagonistic, 14, 36
  arc, 12
  autonomic, 14
  conditioned, 14
  crossed, 14
  postural, 14
  subcutaneous, 14, 85
  superficial, 14
  unconditioned, 14
relaxation, 75, 80, 81, 87
  of the muscles, 111
  techniques, 31, 32
respiratory passages, 93
rheumatoid arthritis, 75, 127, 129

Samilson, Robert, 127
Scholl, Dr, 128
sciatic nerve, 44, 49, 53
sciatica, 116
Shizuoka University, 133
shoulders, 50, 64
  blades, 50
  injury to, 116
  joints, 116
sinuses, 43, 112, 116
skin, as indication of health, 85
  dry, 85, 111, 112, 116
  eruptions, 116
  pigmentation, unnatural, 114, 116
sluggishness, mental, 115
'solar breathing', 54-5
solar plexus, 35, 36, 54, 55, 93-4, 111
The Solar Plexus, 94
spine, 49
spleen, 45, 102, 106
stimulus, 13, 17
stomach, 45, 112
Stone, Dr Randolph, 17
Stopfel, Eunice Ingham, 19, 76, 85, 94, 107, 123
'stretching bones', 31, 32
sunburn, 128
sympathetic nervous system, 93, 94, 111

Taber's Cyclopedic Medical Dictionary, 93
technique, 23-6
tension, 80, 85, 98, 114
testes, 111
testicle, 50
Texas Medical Centre, 133
thoracic cavity, 101
  duct, 106
throat, sore, 111
  tickling in, 113
thymus, 106
thyroid, 85, 112
thyroid-related area, 37, 38
Today's Health, 127
tonsils, 106

underweight, 117

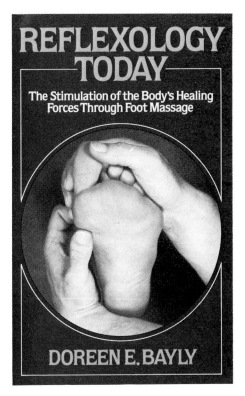

REFLEXOLOGY TODAY

The Stimulation of the Body's Healing Forces Through Foot Massage

DOREEN E. BAYLY

REFLEXOLOGY TODAY
THE STIMULATION OF THE BODY'S HEALING FORCES THROUGH FOOT MASSAGE

Doreen E. Bayly. *Charts & photos.* A reliable guide to the theory and practice of reflexology — the art of restoring the body to health through special massage techniques applied to the feet. Designed as a reference tool for those in doubt about how to treat certain conditions, the book discusses zones and cross reflexes, structure of the feet, how to give a treatment, disorders to be treated through the big toe, arthritis, female irregularities, etc. Includes case histories of author's patients.

REFLEX ZONE
THERAPY
OF THE FEET

A Textbook for Therapists

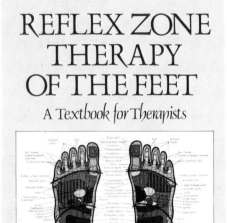

An authoritative guide to treatment

Hanne Marquardt

REFLEX ZONE THERAPY
OF THE FEET
A MANUAL FOR THERAPISTS

Hanne Marquardt. *Illustrated.* First English edition of an authoritative manual by a noted German exponent of reflex zone massage. The book constitutes a reliable guide to diagnosis and includes guidelines for treating specific diseases. *Includes:* The concept of reflex zones; Positioning the patient; The grip-sequence; Common causes of foot complaints; Interpretation of abnormal reflex zones on the feet; Course of treatment; Emollients and 'foot-aids'; Reflex zones of the nervous system; Causal reflex zones.